Wilton Mitsunari Takeshita

The relationship between the golden ratio and facial aesthetics in orthodontics

Wilton Mitsunari Takeshita

The relationship between the golden ratio and facial aesthetics in orthodontics

The golden ratio in dentistry and its evaluation in relation to facial aesthetics in orthodontics

ScienciaScripts

Imprint
Any brand names and product names mentioned in this book are subject to trademark, brand or patent protection and are trademarks or registered trademarks of their respective holders. The use of brand names, product names, common names, trade names, product descriptions etc. even without a particular marking in this work is in no way to be construed to mean that such names may be regarded as unrestricted in respect of trademark and brand protection legislation and could thus be used by anyone.

Cover image: www.ingimage.com

This book is a translation from the original published under ISBN 978-613-9-69262-0.

Publisher:
Sciencia Scripts
is a trademark of
Dodo Books Indian Ocean Ltd. and OmniScriptum S.R.L publishing group

120 High Road, East Finchley, London, N2 9ED, United Kingdom
Str. Armeneasca 28/1, office 1, Chisinau MD-2012, Republic of Moldova, Europe
Printed at: see last page
ISBN: 978-620-8-13072-5

Authors:

DDS, MsD and PhD. Wilton Mitsunari Takeshita - Professor
Adjunct Professor, Department of Dentistry, Federal University of Sergipe,
Brazil

DDS, MsD and PhD and Titular. Edmundo Médici Filho - Retired Professor,
São José dos Campos School of Dentistry - Júlio de Mesquita Filho Paulista
State University

Co-authors:

DDS. Francielle Santos de Santana - Master's student in Dentistry,
Postgraduate Programme in Dentistry, Federal University of Sergipe, Brazil.

DDS, MsD, PhD and Full Professor. Júlio Cezar de Melo Castilho - Retired
Professor, São José dos Campos School of Dentistry - Júlio de Mesquita
Filho Paulista State University.

SUMMARY

Introduction: Beauty is linked to proportionality and this constant proportion gives us the impression of guiding the growth, harmony, reproduction and stability of forms in nature, which has been verified throughout history by scholars such as philosophers, mathematicians, sculptors, painters, architects and orthodontists. Pythagoras, a maths scholar, established proportions based on the standards of beauty and aesthetic harmony, known as the golden ratio. From this thought comes the fact that the golden ratio is used in the assessment of craniofacial structures with the aim of generating an individualised analysis, bringing to each individual proportions obtained on the basis of their own measurements. **Objective: To** present the golden ratio in dentistry and to verify the relationship between the golden ratio and facial aesthetics before and after orthodontic treatment using lateral cephalometric radiographs and frontal and lateral photographs. **Materials and Methods:** Lateral cephalometric radiographs and frontal and lateral photographs of 67 individuals before and after orthodontic treatment were used. A cephalometric programme was developed in Delphi 7.0, containing the cephalometric analysis of this research study. **Conclusions:** In Group 1 (improvement after orthodontic treatment), the A-PogA/1S-C1MS, Ena-Enp/V1S-C1MS and V1S-C1MS/C1MS-DM16 ratios differed in a statistically significant way when comparing before and after orthodontic treatment. The V1S- C1MS/C1MS-DM16 ratio was not golden before treatment and became golden after treatment. In group 2 (no improvement after treatment) only the N- Ena/V1S-DM16 ratio differed in a statistically significant way when comparing before and after treatment. The A-Pog/V1S-DM16 ratio was golden before treatment and was no longer golden after treatment.

KEYWORDS: Cephalometry; photography; golden ratio; orthodontics.

CONTENTS

CHAPTER 1   4

CHAPTER 2   7

CHAPTER 3   13

CHAPTER 4   21

CHAPTER 5   47

CHAPTER 6   54

CHAPTER 7   64

CHAPTER 8   74

CHAPTER 9   85

CHAPTER 1

INTRODUCTION

Human beings have always attached great importance to facial harmony - in other words, beauty. Great civilisations, such as the Egyptians and the Greeks, as well as Renaissance artists, including Michelangelo, demonstrated their appreciation and concern for beauty through endless works of art (PECK & PECK[74] ,1970). However, when it comes to beauty, the ability to recognise beauty is innate, and there is an individual preference with cultural influence so that trying to translate it into objective and defined therapeutic goals is very difficult (SUGUINO *et al.*[TM3] ,1996).

Beauty is linked to proportionality and this constant proportion gives us the impression of guiding the growth, harmony, reproduction and stability of forms in nature, which has been verified throughout history by scholars such as philosophers, mathematicians, sculptors, painters, architects and orthodontists (GIL & MEDICI FILHO[32] , 2002; MARTINS[58] , 2003).

Pythagoras, a maths scholar, established proportions based on standards of beauty and aesthetic harmony. It has been called the golden ratio by many scholars, the divine ratio by Paccioli, the divine section by Kepler and in this research project it will be called the golden ratio (BAUM[10] , 1966; GIL & MEDICI FILHO[32] , 2002; BAKER & WOODS[8] , 2001).

The golden ratio is generated from the proportionality expressed by the number 1.618033... (usually used 1.618), obtained by applying the following formula: $qj = (1+5) / 2$. We will use the Greek character cp(fi) to determine the proportionality ratio. (generally used 1.618), obtained by applying the following formula: $qj = (1+5^{1/2}) / 2$. We will use the Greek character cp(fi) to determine the ratio of proportionality, as Phidias was a Greek sculptor who made extensive use of the divine proportion. In simplified terms, we can say that the golden ratio is explained as follows: by dividing a line asymmetrically, a proportion is maintained such that the larger segment is to the smaller one as the sum of the two is to the larger one (Figure 1).

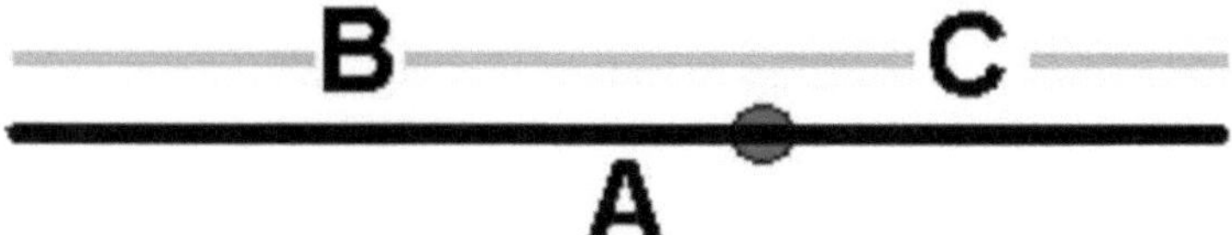

FIGURE 1 - Description of the golden ratio, line segment divided into mean and extreme ratio: A=1.618; B=1; C=0.618. B/C=C/B =1.618[54]

This relationship can also be seen in the Fibonacci series, where one number is the sum of the two previous ones and dividing one number by the previous one results in the golden number 1.618 (Figure 2).

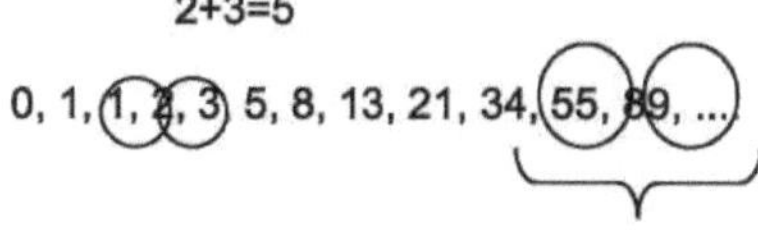

FIGURA 2   - If we divide 89 by 55, the result will be 1.618 and if we add 2 to 3, the result will be 5. This establishes a sequence[25] .

This series can also be observed in nature, for example in the distribution of petals in flowers, in the reproduction of animals, in the shape of animals and in human beings.

In the field of psychology, various studies have been carried out to assess human aesthetic preference, finding that attraction and appreciation of beauty seem to be related to structures that are in golden ratio. In this respect, Rickets[88] (1982) states: "The golden ratio seems to have some marvellous and unique property. It is the quality that for some reason attracts attention and is emphasised in the limbic system as beautiful, harmonious and balanced."

The study of this subject is of interest to a wide variety of areas: Orthodontics, Oral and Maxillofacial Surgery, Dentistry and Plastic Surgery. Rickets[88] , 1982; Amoric[4] , 1995; Gil & Mediei Filho[32] , 2002, when carrying out cephalometric analyses, proved the existence of the golden ratio in some measurements. Therefore, when orthodontic planning, it is extremely important to consider not only the patient's occlusal balance, but also their aesthetic preferences, analysing the facial qualities of symmetry, harmony and proportion (WUERPEL[113] , 1932; RIEDEL[89] , 1950; PECK & PECK[74] , 1970; RICKETS[88] , 1982). In addition, it is worth emphasising that harmonious and beautiful faces provide individuals with high self-esteem and excellent psycho-social interaction (HOWELLS & SHAW[36] , 1985; PEERLING *etal.*[75] , 1995; KÕLLER[44] , 2006).

From this thought comes the fact that the use of the golden ratio in the assessment of craniofacial structures aims to generate an individualised analysis, bringing to each individual proportions obtained on the basis of their own measurements, and not those obtained from the population average and that knowing the structures in golden ratio can, for example, return to patients treated surgically and orthodontically, the measurements that are most harmonious to them and not those that occur in the population average.

The purpose of this research project was to speed up the transfer of research data directly to statistical analysis programmes, since a computer programme called Aurea Ceph was developed and therefore does not use existing cephalometry programmes on the market. The Aurea Ceph programme makes it possible to apply the golden ratio in the assessment of lateral cephalometric radiographs. The software was developed based on a programming algorithm that will be explained later.

As for photography, it is undoubtedly a great auxiliary tool for research, diagnosis and planning, as long as it is obtained in a standardised way, allowing it to be reproduced at different times and spaced out, with fidelity and reliability (BISHARA ef a/.[13] , 1995).

The purpose of this study was to verify the relationship between the golden ratio and facial aesthetics before and after orthodontic treatment, using lateral cephalometric radiographs and frontal and lateral photographs.

CHAPTER 2

The golden ratio

In mathematical terms, a proportion is an equality between ratios. A ratio is the result of a division, a fractional distribution. When this distribution leaves no leftovers, it is said to be exact. When two ratios are equal, they are said to be proportional (TAVARES *et al.*[TM5] 2006). When we have a line segment with ends A and B, we can determine a point D on this segment by dividing it into a mean and an extreme ratio. The aim is to find a point D between A and B such that the ratio between segment AB and segment AD is <P (1.61803) (Figure 3) (SODRÉ & TOFFOLI", 2003).

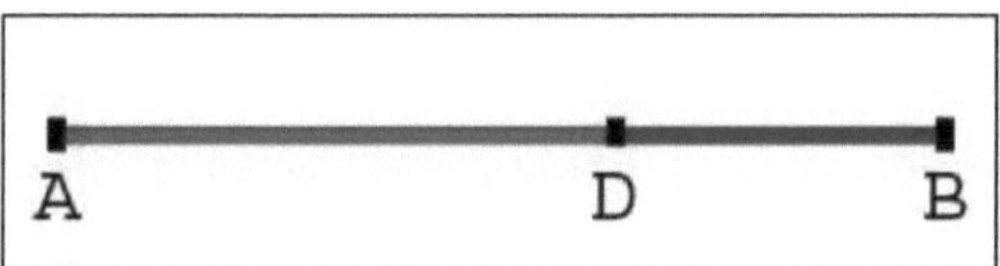

$$\frac{AB}{AD} = \frac{AD}{DB} = \phi = \frac{1 + \sqrt{5}}{2}$$

FIGURE 3 - This shows that the longest segment AD is 1.618033... times the length of the shortest segment DB[90].

Two different quantities, and only two, can provide a continuous proportion. If the quantities are a and b, their sum a+b gives the required term: a+b/a = a/b, which is a famous proportion and is based on the golden number, which is obtained when a/b=1.618 (Figure 4) (SOUZA *et al:*[°°] 2006).

$$\frac{a+b}{a} = \frac{a}{b} \quad \rightarrow \quad 1 + \frac{b}{a} = \frac{a}{b}$$

Se $\dfrac{a}{b} = x$ então $1 + \dfrac{1}{x} = x$ Ou

$$x^2 - x - 1 = 0$$

Verififica-se que $x_{,} = \dfrac{1+\sqrt{5}}{2}$ e $x_{,,} = \dfrac{1-\sqrt{5}}{2}$

$\dfrac{1+\sqrt{5}}{2} = 1{,}618034$ é chamado o Número de Ouro

Se $a+b = 1$, assim $\dfrac{a+b}{a} = \dfrac{a}{b} = x$

$$\frac{a}{b} = 1{,}618034 \, , \quad \frac{b}{a} = 0{,}618034$$

FIGURE 4 - Mathematical equation for obtaining the golden number[61] .

The study of the golden ratio, according to Herodotus, a Greek historian, began in ancient times. He came to this conclusion when Egyptian priests told him that the dimensions of the pyramid of Giseh were built according to the following relationship: the area of the square, whose side is the height of the great pyramid, was equal to the area of the triangular face. A very simple algebra can be used to show that the ratio between the height of a triangular face and half the length of the base is in golden ratio (GIL[30] , 1999) (Figure 5).

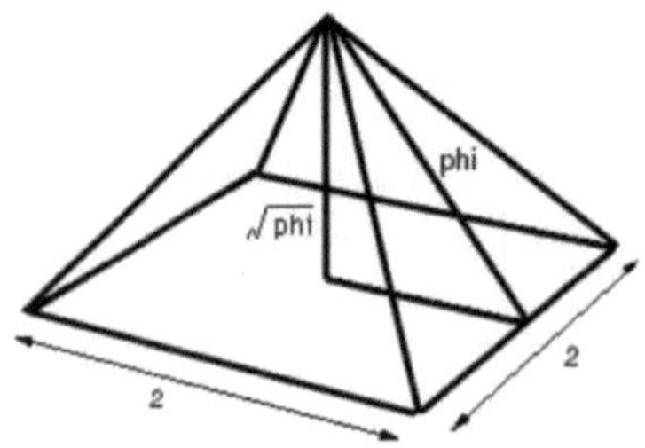

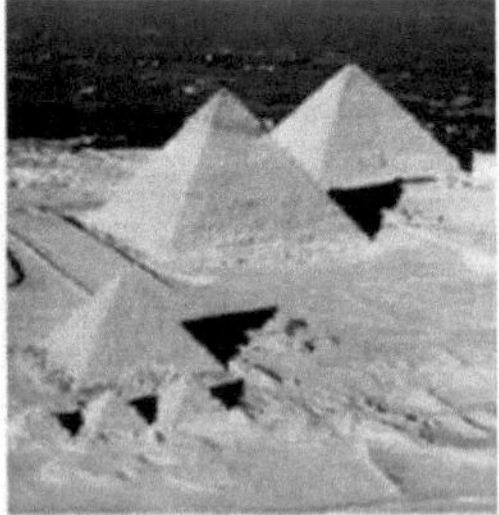

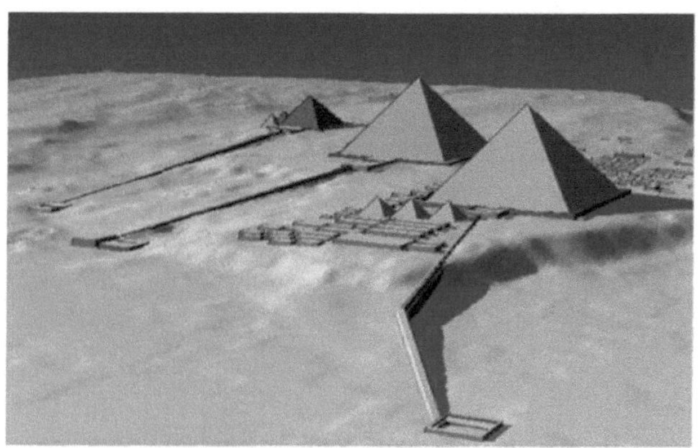

FIGURE 5 - Diagram showing the construction of the Pyramids of Giseh.[68]

The Egyptians considered the golden number to be sacred and of the utmost importance in their religion. They used it to build temples and tombs for the dead, because they considered that if this didn't happen, the temple might not please the Gods or the soul wouldn't be able to reach the Alem. In the temple of Dendara, for example, inside there is a spiral staircase, very similar in shape to the golden spiral, an applied form of the golden ratio. The Egyptians also used the golden number in their writing system (RANULFO[84] , 2005).

Euclid of Alexandria (365 BC - 300 BC) was also of great importance to the history of geometry. He developed the theory of the golden ratio, where two numbers (X and Y, for example) are in golden ratio if the ratio of the smaller of the two to the larger is equal to the larger of the sum of the two (i.e. X/Y = Y/X+Y). This ratio establishes a golden ratio, where it can be analysed that basically everything found in nature is inscribed in this ratio, be it the human body, a hive of bees, a starfish, a shell, etc (Figure 6) (FERRAZ[26] , 2004).

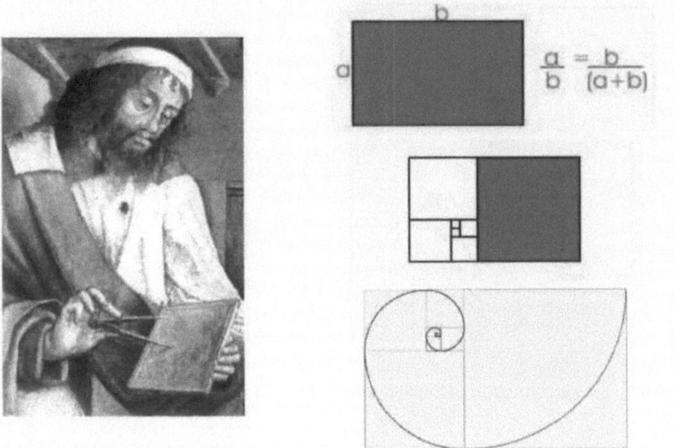

FIGURE 6 - Euclid of Alexandria and his reasoning on the golden number. The golden rectangle can be divided into smaller squares and rectangles (always golden). What's more, if we draw a quarter of a circle around each square inside the golden rectangle, we get the golden spiral. Below are examples of applications of the golden ratio to constructions[21] .

In the 5th and 4th centuries BC, Greek sculpture reached its peak. The most famous Greek sculptor of this period, Phidias, built one of the greatest Greek temples, the Parthenon (430-440 BC). The ground plan of the Parthenon shows that the temple was built on the basis of the golden rectangle, and the golden ratio can be seen in the distances between the columns and also in the interior spaces (Figure 7) (PETRONZELI[76] , 2005).

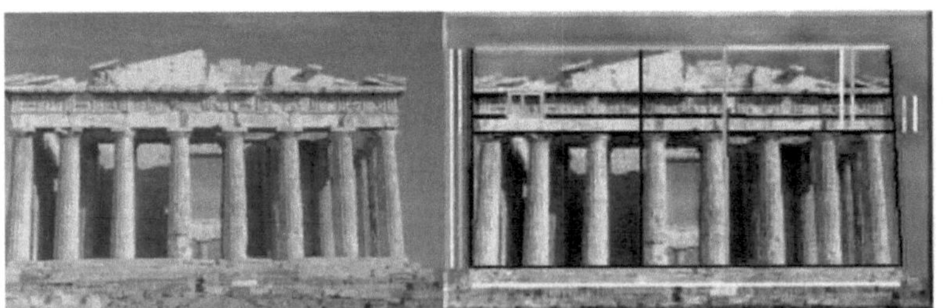

FIGURA 7   - The structure of the Parthenon shows that the façade is a golden rectangle.[68]

The Renaissance sparked a new interest in ancient knowledge and revived the study of Pythagorean proportions. A study by Leonardo Da Vinci shows the relationships of proportion in the human face (Figure 8)

(SOUZA *et al.*[100] 2006).

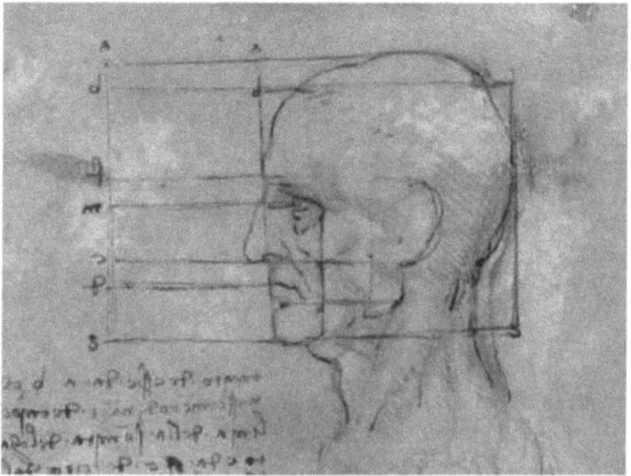

FIGURA 8   - In Leonardo Da Vinci's drawing, the artist superimposed on the sketch a square divided into rectangles, some of which are similar to the golden rectangle[91] .

In the Renaissance, the teachings of Vitruvius gained great importance. The anthropometric data he presented was drawn by Leonardo Da Vinci in his famous work "L'Uomo di Vitruvio" (Vitruvian Man).(Figure 9)(LOPES FILHO & SILVA[51] , 2006)

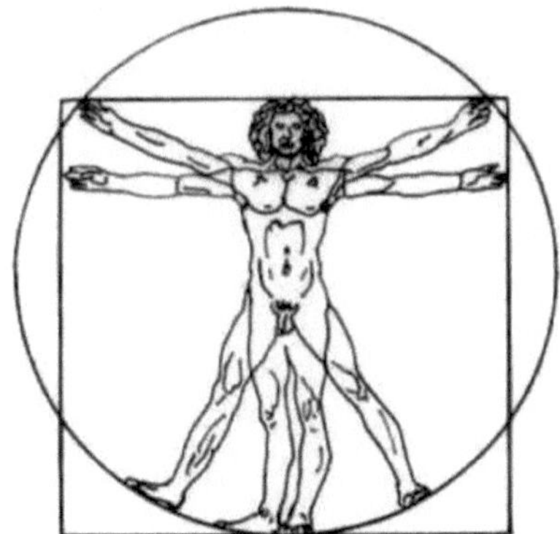

FIGURA 9   - Leonardo Da Vinci exhaustively studied the proportions of the human form, resulting in the famous drawing in which the human body is placed in the ideal shape of a circle and in the perfect proportions of a square.[45]

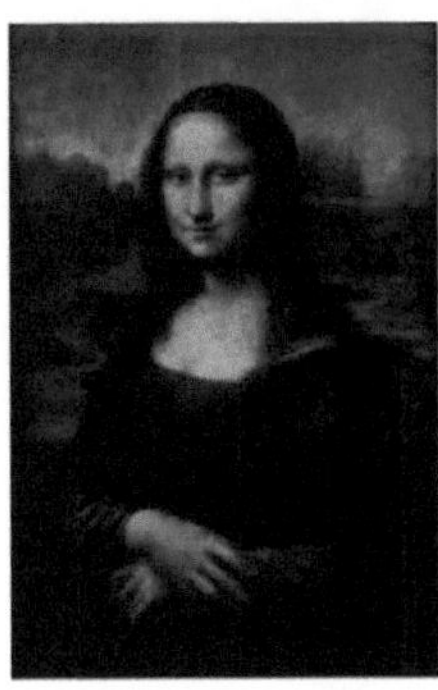

FIGURA 10   - Leonardo da Vinci used golden ratio to paint the Mona Lisa, one of his most remarkable works. At various points in the work, such as the relationship between her torso and head, or between the elements of her face, they appear in golden ratio[21] .

CHAPTER 3

Golden ratio in nature and the Fibonacci numbers

In 1202, the greatest European mathematician of the Middle Ages, Fibonacci, completed his book *Liber Abaci*, which influenced many mathematicians to use the Hindu-Arabic system, which he introduced to Europe, which until then had used Roman numerals (GIL[30] , 1999). This book describes the Fibonacci series (mentioned above), which can be observed in various ways and also through the illustrations provided by Jefferson[41] (2003), Knott^OOS), Levin[47] (2003) and Netto[67] (2003).

For example, Knott[47] (2003) reported that by associating this with general biology, we can see that rabbits reproduce in golden ratio (Fibonacci series). Assuming that a pair of rabbits, a female and a male, are placed in a fenced field and that they become sexually mature in one month, then at the end of the second month the female can produce a new pair of rabbits. Assuming that our rabbits never die and that the female always produces a new pair (a female and a male) every month. Then we will have:

a) from the first month onwards, they cross, but they remain just a pair;

b) at the end of the second month, the original female produces a new pair, so now there are two pairs;

c) at the end of the third month the original female produces a second pair, making three pairs;

d) the female born in the second month produces her first pair, making five pairs.

e) the sequence formed will then be: 0, 1, 1, 2 , 3, 5, 8, 13, 21, 34, ... infinitely.

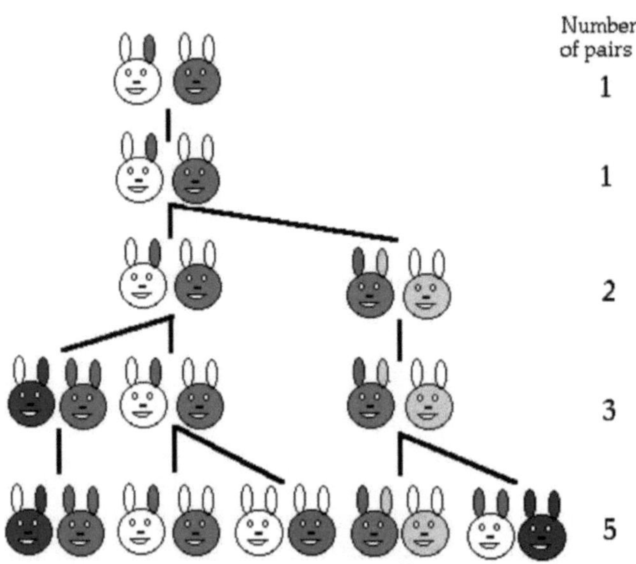

FIGURE 11 - Diagram of the rabbit family tree.[90]

We can also see in the *spira nautilus* snail that its spiral shape can be demonstrated using the Fibonacci Spiral. It can be described as follows using the series 1, 1, 2, 3, 5, 8, 13, 21, 34, ... considering the first square of size 1, one on top of the other (1+1=2, 2+1=3, 3+2=5, 3+5=8, 5+8=13, 8+13=21, and so on, we then build a spiral and if we want to add squares around the figure, with each next square having the measure of the sum of the two previous ones, we get the spiral of the size we want (MEISNER[60] , 2003).

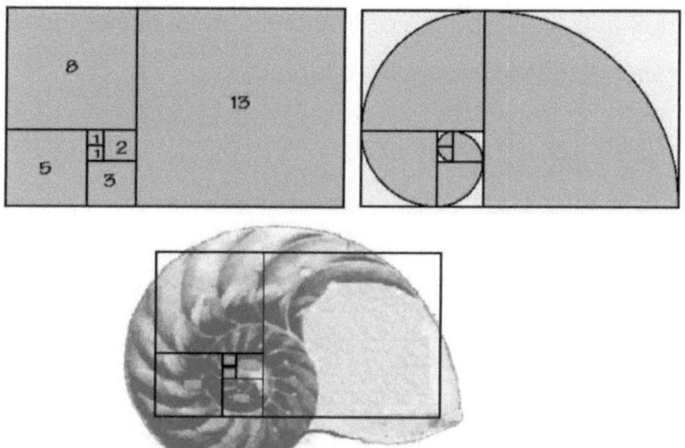

FIGURA 12   - Fibonacci spiral. These drawings show that we can build a spiral by joining quarters of circles, one in each new square. This *spiral* is similar to that of the *spira nautilus* snail.[90]

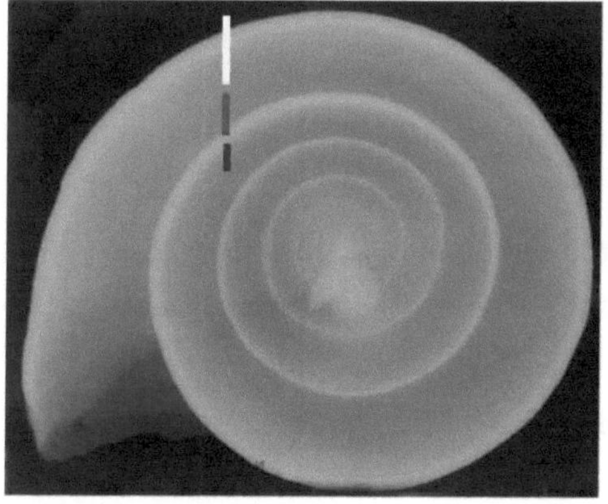

FIGURA 13   - Radiograph of the snail's shell taken in Radiology. We can still see the golden ratio in the shape of the animals:

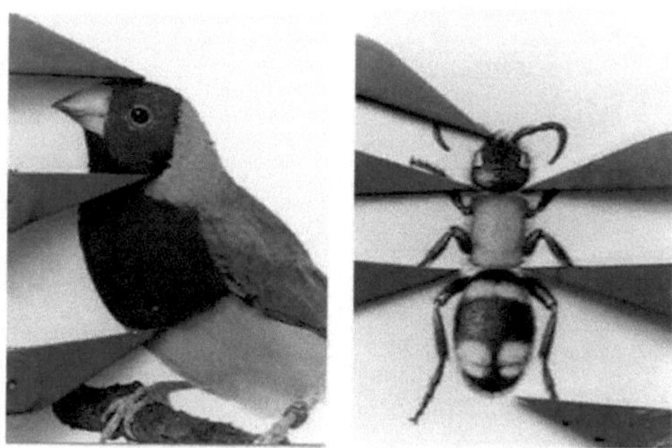

FIGURA 14   - Golden ratio in the shape of animals.[41]

If we also look at the distribution of branches, most plants follow the pattern below. The branches divide at regular intervals.

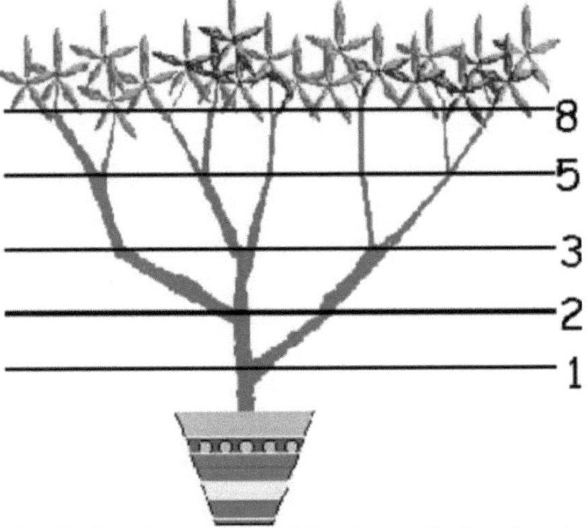

FIGURA 15   - Suppose that it takes two months for a branch on a plant to be strong enough to support a division with a new branch. If a new branch is born every month, we'll have a plant like this.[90]

The Fibonacci series can be seen in the distribution of seeds in the centre of flowers. In the diagram of the core of a sunflower or daisy below, you can see that the seeds form spirals that turn to the right and left, totalling 34 spirals. The same happens with seeds in nature. No matter how big the core of the flower, the seeds are packed evenly, not piled up in the centre and not too scattered around the edges, and it can be seen that they are distributed according to the Fibonacci numbers.

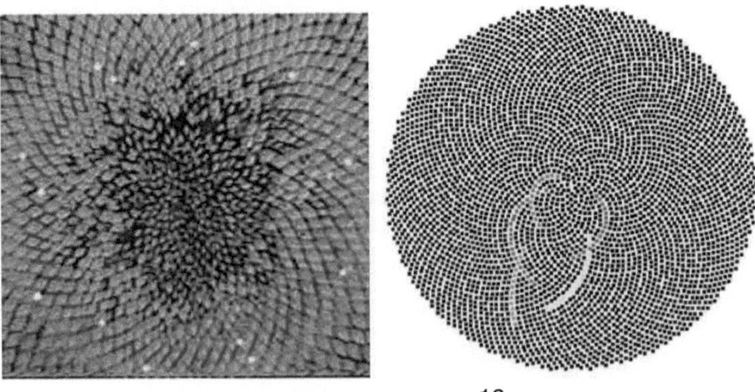

FIGURE 16 - Schematic of the distribution of sunflower seeds in a spiral pattern.[13]

Meisner[6] °(2003), reported that the golden ratio can also be observed in the shape of the ear, with the Fibonacci Spiral being an applied form of the golden ratio (Figure 17). The author also reports that in the echocardigram, the heartbeat is in golden ratio (Figure 18). DNA spirals are in golden ratio (Figure 19).

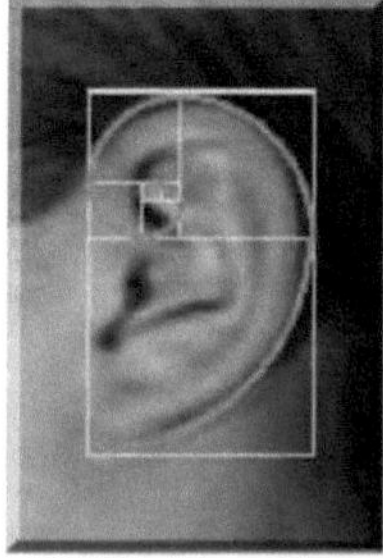

FIGURA 17   - Shape of the ear describing the Fibonacci Spiral.[54]

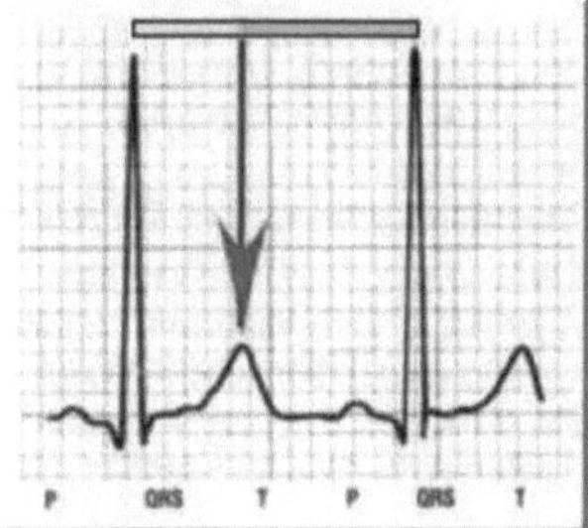

FIGURA 18   - Golden ratio echocardiogram.[54]

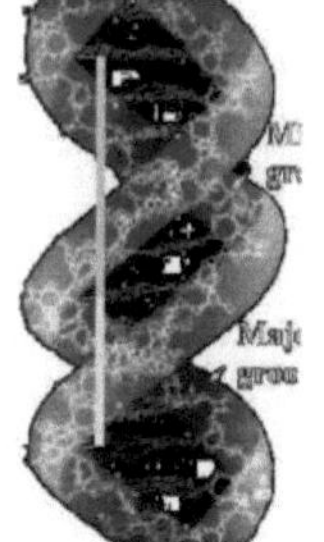

FIGURA 19   - The spirals of DNA are in golden ratio.[54]

In his studies, Marquadt[56] (2006) developed a mask based on the golden ratio. According to the author, this is a tool for dentistry and plastic surgery. To make the mask, the author starts from a sectioned line based on the golden number, doubling the largest segment and joining the distances gives an obtuse golden triangle, doubling the smallest segment gives an obtuse triangle. If you join two obtuse golden triangles with an acute golden triangle, you get a golden pentagon. Superimposing two golden pentagons produces the Golden Decagon, the basis for creating the Marquadt mask. The author also reports on a technique for superimposing an individual's photo on the mask in order to assess the individual's facial proportions (Figure 20).

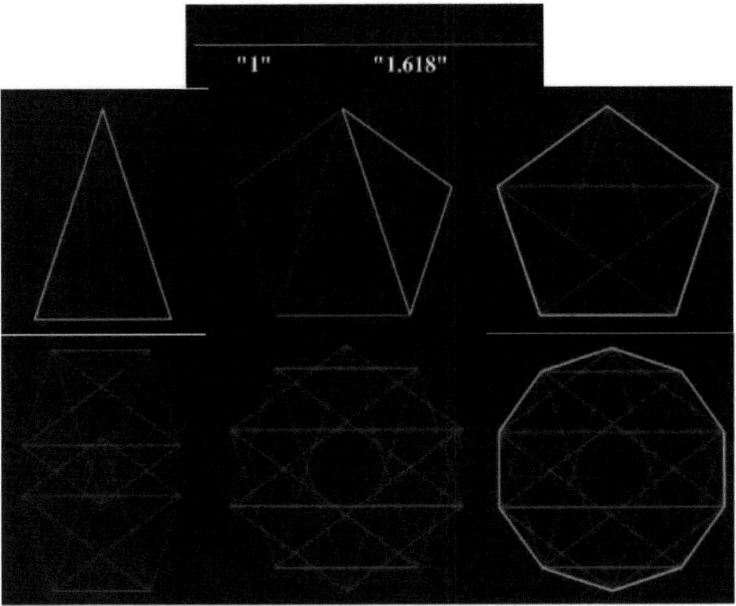

FIGURE 20 - Diagram showing the formation of the Golden Decagon.[50]

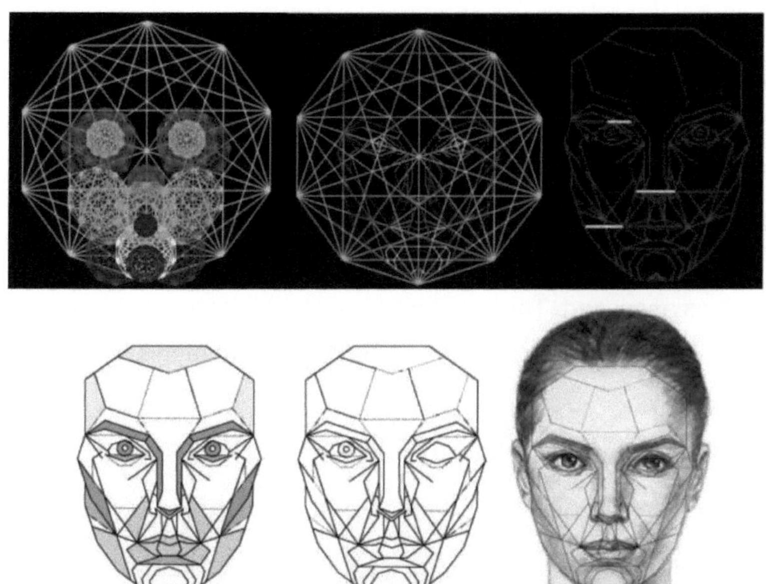

FIGURE 21 - The Marquadt mask is formed using the Golden Decagon.[50]

The following is a demonstration of the applicability of the mask created by Marquadt, especially in terms of its relationship with aesthetics. In Figure 22 we can see the mask superimposed on two different faces, and we can see that the mask does not fit on the non-harmonious face.

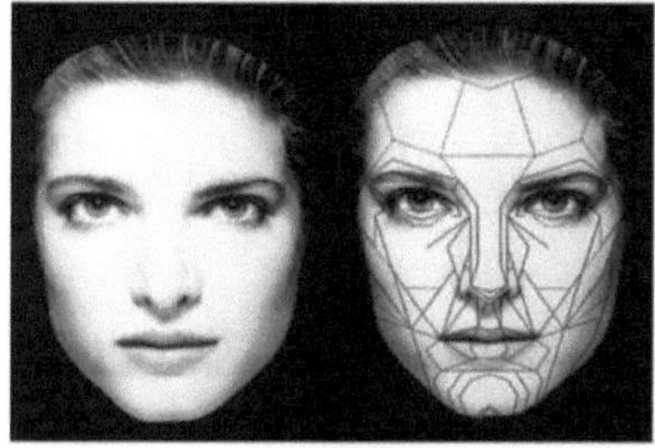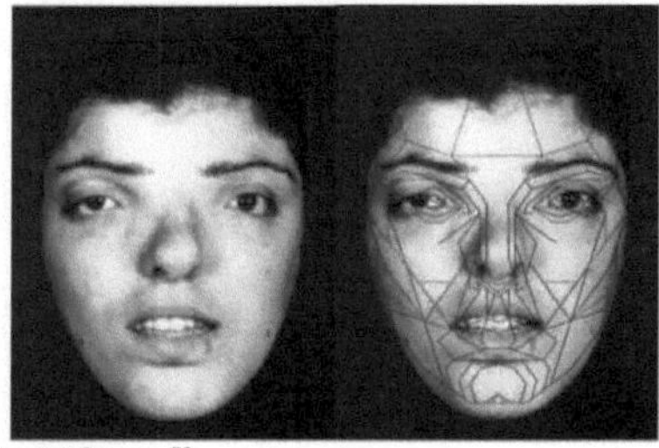

FIGURE 22 - Overlaying the mask on two different faces.[50]

Bertollo *et al*™ (2008) investigated whether this proportion manifests itself in the faces of people selected by evaluators, using the criterion of beauty. The initial sample consisted of 104 people, previously selected and separated into groups M (male) and F (female), and two photographic records (A and B) were taken of each participant. Photographs (frontal and lateral) were obtained from photographic record A and submitted for examination by a group of assessors. Once the values had been assigned, the subjects who would make up the final sample were identified: subgroups M1 and F1 (10 people with the highest numerical value) and M2 and F2 (10 people with the lowest numerical value), totalling a final sample of 80 photographs (frontal and lateral) from photographic record B. The actual facial analysis was carried out. The data obtained was compared with the Divine Proportion, observing it in only two of the proportions assessed. Thus, it can be said that the Divine Proportion is not associated with the perception of beauty in the context of this research.

CHAPTER 4

The golden ratio and facial aesthetics

In 1932, Wuerpel[113] emphasised the importance of beauty for human beings by stating that beauty is a vital force in the development of our lives. He also reported that beauty is the finest expression of human emotion and therefore difficult to define in words. He also questioned the possibility of all ages, races and individuals, over time, accepting the same laws of feeling, emotion and expression. By evaluating human behaviour in the face of concepts of beauty, from the Stone Age to the present day, he concluded that past reactions to these concepts have changed over time.

Wuerpel[114] reported in 1937 that the orthodontic professional's ultimate goal should not only be to restore normal occlusion, but also to achieve the best facial appearance, i.e. to achieve facial balance and harmony.

In his article on aesthetics and its relationship with orthodontic treatment, Riedel[89] (1950) reported on the primary objectives of orthodontic treatment: improving function, improving aesthetics and maintaining these improvements. The author used lateral cephalometric radiographs, plaster models, frontal and lateral photographs taken of children and adults clinically with normal occlusion and cases of orthodontically treated individuals. Cephalometric tracings and the contour of the profile line were obtained for all the radiographs. The profiles were evaluated by 88 orthodontists who classified the profile as "good" or "bad". The following conclusions were reached:

a) opinions on the profiles were uniform;

b) there was a difference in the skeletal and dental patterns of individuals with a "good" and "bad" profile, indicating that the aesthetic relationship and facial harmony interacted with the dental skeletal pattern.

Ricketts[85] reported in 1957 that aesthetics should be one of the objectives of orthodontic treatment, which is why there is a need to know the concepts of balance and facial harmony. According to the author, the term balance corresponds to a correct proportion between the facial elements and facial harmony corresponds to the adaptation between these elements.

Riedel[90] , in 1957, when studying facial aesthetics, observed that the population's concept of facial beauty coincided with the cephalometric standards determined by orthodontics. To determine the concepts of aesthetics, he obtained lateral cephalometric radiographs of 30 young women chosen as princesses for the Seattle Sea Fair and found that their skeletal pattern was similar to those pre-established by orthodontists, concluding that the soft profile is only slightly related to the bone profile and dental structures.

Burstone[19] (1958) used lateral cephalometric radiographs and photographs of forty individuals with harmonious facial features chosen by a group of three artists from the Herron Institute of Arts in Indianapolis. He concluded that appearance is one of the fundamental functions of the face, which, in turn, is not only important for digestion, breathing or phonation, but also has an extreme influence on the psychological well-being and acceptance of the individual in the social environment in which they live. Thus, the notion of profile differs from person to person, depending on the racial and ethnic group to which they belong, and soft tissue cannot be assessed solely through a study of the skeletal pattern, as this may be inadequate for assessing disharmony in the facial profile.

Goldsman[33] , in 1959, set out to research the dento-skeletal model of adult Caucasians considered to have excellent faces, and submitted front and profile photos of 160 Caucasian individuals between the ages of 15 and 36, to be assessed by a jury of artists from the Buffalo Art Institute in New York and the Herron Art Institute in Indianapolis, who selected the fifty photographs with the excellent faces. All had Class I and only one had received orthodontic treatment. Surprisingly, the jury was unanimous in their choice of subjects, which led them to conclude that artists are more liberal in their conception of facial harmony than orthodontists who have preconceived and even harmful ideas of what constitutes ideal facial aesthetics.

Baum[10] , in 1966, reported in his article that the progression of changes certainly follows a model that can be measured and classified for scientific purposes; each patient has their own individuality. Orthodontists cannot practice their profession "through numbers" and emphasised that patients are not the average of a group. Thus, there is individuality, integrity and these characteristics are related to beauty. According to the author, the individual combinations of facial features certainly have the culture as a whole accepting the representation of beauty. He also reported that the concept of facial aesthetics is variable and represented by a set of characteristics inherent to culture, time and fashion. In order to analyse changes in the facial profile during orthodontic treatment, the author carried out a longitudinal study on 23 males and 21 females who had dental malocclusion and normal occlusion at the end of orthodontic treatment. He concluded that the dental arch of males retracts and the profile of females remains essentially the same. He also found that the
growth period in males was longer and more protracted than in females.

Peck & Peck[74] , 1970, surveyed studies on facial aesthetics, from prehistoric times to the date of their work, including the Egyptians, Greeks, Romans and Renaissance artists, in which the quote stands out, according to philosophers who believed that beautiful creations respected certain geometric laws, since true beauty manifests harmony. As harmony was the due observance of proportions, it seems reasonable that these proportions were fixed quantities. The authors stated that art had been aiming for beauty, proportion and harmony for over five thousand years. They studied 52 young adult individuals selected as part of an aesthetically pleasing population, as it included professional models, beauty pageant winners and artists, all with facial attractiveness. By analysing cephalometrics, they concluded that the public preferred a fuller profile with more protruding dento-facial relationships, when compared to the usual cephalometric patterns. They stated that orthodontists should treat their patients not to satisfy their own concepts of beauty, but those of society. They emphasised the importance of aesthetic preferences when planning orthodontic treatment, analysing the facial qualities of symmetry, harmony and proportion.

When it comes to the golden ratio in human beings, in 1970 Torres[107] , gave a history of the golden ratio, citing Pythagoras, Paccioli, Leonardo da Vinci, Alberti, Euclid and Fibonacci. And he describes the presence of the golden ratio in human beings. On the body and face:

a) the navel divides the total height of the body in golden ratio;

b) the arm extended at the side of the body divides in golden ratio, at the height of the longest finger;

c) the bones of the body are in golden ratio: metacarpals and phalanges (Figure 23);

d) distance between the subnasal-labial commissure cp commissure- gnathion;

e) pupil line-nose tip cp nose tip-commissure;

f) ear canal-commissure cp commissure-gnathium (divides the mandible into body and ramus).

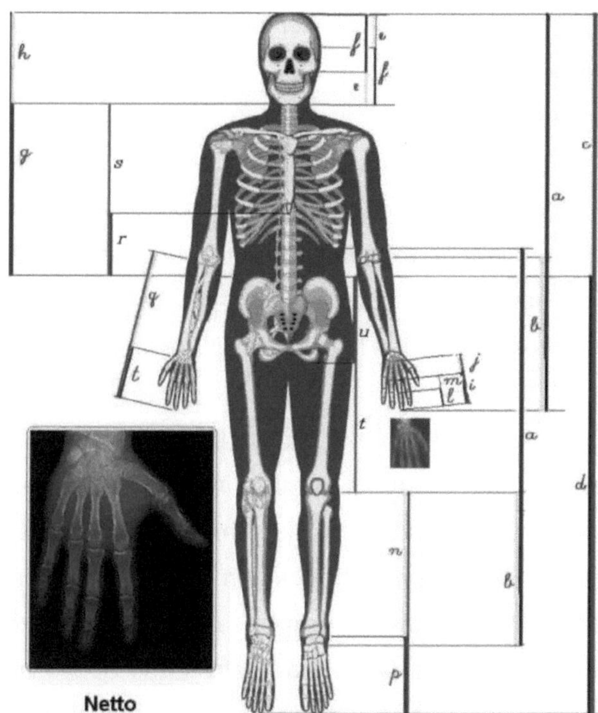

FIGURE 23 - Golden proportions of the human body.[61]

In 1972, Rickets[86] demonstrated in detail the direction of mandibular growth. The author carried out a study using forty frontal and lateral cephalometric radiographs of subjects aged five, eight and 13 years; twenty subjects had normal occlusion, the rest had Class II occlusion. A computerised study of 362 cephalometric measurements was carried out over a period of five years. In the mandibles of individuals with normal occlusion, an arch growth was observed, which described a logarithmic spiral, which represents an applied form of the golden number.

In 1976, Benjafield[11] studied the aesthetic preference for golden rectangles. The rectangles were presented to 180 individuals, divided into different groups of 15 men and 15 women. Each group had the same presentation conditions. The evaluators had to separate the rectangles they considered most pleasing and then separate the one they liked the most. The individuals tended to favour the larger rectangles over the smaller ones and those close to the golden ratio. He concluded that the golden ratio is still the preferable and most pleasing ratio.

Powell & Rayson[80] (1976) concluded that facial beauty is an open field for scientific research, in which facial changes are studied objectively, but the aesthetic interpretation of the changes remains subjective because there are many different facial types, each of which can present its own variables such as growth, posture, expression, age and changes resulting from treatments carried out.

According to Ghynka[29] , 1977, the human body has several golden ratio measurements. The author reported that he had analysed hundreds of human skeletons and published the results of his measurements. Although the individual measurements vary, and although even the way in which the proportions interrelate can vary, every normal skeleton reveals that it is harmonious. For the author, the skeletons showed details and above all shapes more rigorously than in living man; the body where we have skin, muscle tissue, shows fluctuations that are more difficult to translate into precise measurements. He pointed out that structures with this proportion have an aesthetic and harmonious appearance. She said that when you divide the human body at the navel, when you divide the largest part by the smallest part, you find the golden ratio. Ghynka[29] reported that this relationship is established at the age of 13, and that individuals up to this age do not have their structure in golden ratio, since at birth the navel divides the human body into two equal parts.

Levin[48] in 1978, in his article Dental aesthetics and the golden ratio, reported that geometry has two great treasures: one is the Pythagorean theorem, the other the division of a line into mean and extreme ratio. The author described the application of the golden ratio to dental aesthetics. He observed in a frontal photograph that the width of the upper central incisor was in golden proportion to the width of the upper lateral incisor.

In his 1978 study, Piehl[78] used rectangles with different side size ratios but approximately equal areas, which were presented to one hundred and twenty people to assess their aesthetic preferences for each rectangle. The golden rectangle was the one that people tended to prefer. In addition, rectangles similar to the golden rectangle were also favoured.

Ricketts[87] , in 1981, described the golden ratio applied to various parts of the human body. He reported that the golden ratio can be applied in orthodontic treatment in relation to teeth, bones and soft tissues and also in the planning of oral and maxillofacial surgery and plastic surgery, proposing a treatment with an individualised analysis as opposed to the average measurements of the population. He also mentioned the golden proportions in the dental arch: the width of the upper lateral incisors is in golden proportion to the width of the upper central incisors and the lower central incisors are in golden proportion to the lower central incisors. In his research, he used a sample of thirty individuals with normal occlusion. He described the golden proportions of the face, i.e. the soft tissues, as follows: the width of the wing of the nose, the width of the mouth, the lateral corner of both eyes and the width of the head at the height of the eyebrows are in golden proportion. He also found eight golden ratios in lateral cephalometric radiographs and concluded that the structures of the skull are in golden ratio in the anterior and posterior regions of the skull base.

In 1982, Ricketts[88] described the application of basic maths and the geometric principles of the normal morphology of the structures regularly involved in orthodontics and dentistry, the Fibonacci numbers, the golden rectangle, pentagon analysis and the golden triangle. He suggested that aesthetics could be done in a scientific manner, rather than having to rely on subjective perceptions as was the case in the past. To verify this hypothesis, he randomly selected from a magazine ten frontal photographs of people with various facial types, chosen for their excellent beauty, and of different ethnicities. His sample consisted of seven leucoderms, two xanthoderms and one melanoderm. For the frontal width ratio, i.e. in the horizontal direction, the following points were selected: LN=the lateral edge of the wing of the nose; CH=chilon, a point at the angle of the mouth; LC=a point on the side of the corner of the eyes; NB=a point at the base of the nasal bridge and TS=a point on the lateral edge of the temple at the level of the eyebrow. The following points were selected for the height ratio, i.e. in the vertical direction: TRI=Trichion uppermost point on the forehead contour; EB=point on the lower edge of the upper corner of the eyebrow curve; LC=lateral corner of the eye; AL=upper corner of the alar curve of the nose; St=stomion, selected on the same level as the chilon (CH) on the midline; ME=soft tissue of the chin, lower edge of the chin. The author concluded the following golden ratio relationships for width: LN-LN <p CH-CH, LC-LC 9 CH-CH, LC-LC <p LN-LN and TS-TS <p LC-LC. With regard to height, the following golden ratio relationships were observed: TRI-LC <p LC-ME, LN-ME 9 LN-TRI, LN-LC 9 LN-ME, LC-CH 9 CH-ME, LN-LC 9 CH- ME (Figure 24).

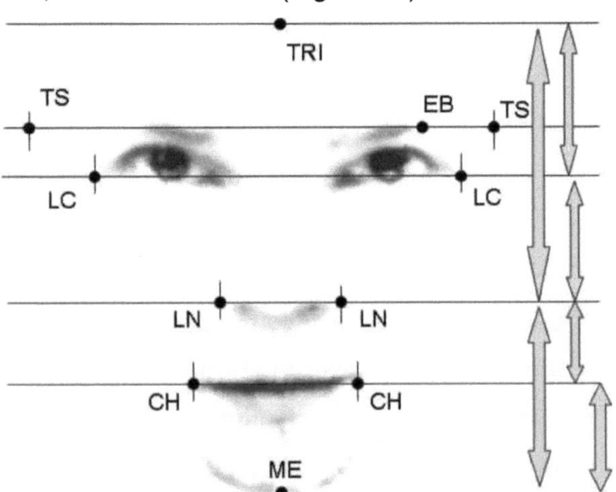

FIGURE 24 - Measurements observed by Ricketts[80] (1982) in golden ratio.

Marinho Filho *et al.*[55] 1982, publicised notions of the golden ratio, trying to adapt aspects of cephalometry to it. The authors reported on the construction of the golden rectangle and its application in radiographic cephalometry.

Barrer & Ghafari[9] , in their 1985 study, described the use of profile silhouette drawing to determine the effects of orthodontic treatment on facial aesthetics. Forty-one individuals with Angle Class II Division 1 malocclusion were used for the sample. One hundred first-year dental students evaluated the profile drawing to determine the most aesthetic faces and classify them as satisfactory or unsatisfactory. The authors concluded that the profile design after treatment was favoured over the design before treatment.

Nakajima & Yanagisawa[65] , in 1985, described the application of the golden ratio described by Ricketts[88] (1982), to elucidate the possible relationship between the sense of beauty and beautiful facial proportion revealed by the faces of Japanese people. Firstly, using Ricketts' methodology[88] (1982), the authors investigated patients with malocclusion. Secondly, to propose which type of face has a beautiful facial proportion from the point of view of Japanese culture. The sample consisted of 34 individuals (six males and 12 females with Class II malocclusion and seven males and nine females with Class III malocclusion). The authors related the face, eyes, nose and mouth. In the studies by Ricketts[88] (1982), the mouth is in golden proportion to the nose. In the case of the Japanese, some measurements were not in proportion. Two possible reasons for this are:

a) the nose is bigger than the mouth;

b) the mouth is small in relation to the nose, however, according to the author it is well known that Japanese mouths are smaller than those of Caucasians.

Nakajima *et al.*[66] published a second article in 1985, following on from their previous work in 1985. In this second article, the authors described the sense of beauty and beautiful facial proportions from the point of view of Japanese culture. Using the methodology employed by Ricketts[88] (1982), the authors selected seven women considered to have beautiful faces. The authors concluded that on the faces of the Japanese they obtained numerical values close to the square root of two. This value can be observed in the construction of temples in Japan, Shitennoji Temple in Namba and Horyuji Temple in Yamato, and can also be seen in the portrait drawing of Prince Shotoku.

Czarnecki *et al.*[23] , 1993, in a study on facial profile balance, used a sample of male and female individuals, distributed in three series with seven profiles in each and evaluated by 545 professionals. The profiles varied according to the silhouettes formed by the lips, nose and chin. For men, the straight profile was accepted as beautiful and harmonious and for women, the slightly convex profile was found. They concluded that there is a great deal of agreement on the facial profile and that there is a great deal of agreement between observers on the most attractive and least attractive profiles, even in cases where different groups of observers were asked, for example laypeople and orthodontists. This makes us think once again that there is a conception of facial balance that is common to all.

Mew[61] , in 1993, began his article by stating that facial beauty is largely responsible for generating emotions in human beings, having a fundamental influence on the relationship between individuals of opposite sexes, which is to attract them to each other. In his research, the author drew five faces and then randomly presented them to 105 adults aged between 16 and 60. In the most attractive face, the zygomatic prominence was more convex anteriorly. For the least attractive face, the zygomatic prominence was more retruded and flat. The author concluded that small characteristics can modify appearance and, consequently, facial aesthetics.

In 1993, Preston[81] studied the golden ratio and its application to dental aesthetics. The author proposed evaluating the golden ratio relationship between the size of the upper central incisor and the lower central incisor. Orthodontic models of 58 second-year students at the University of Southern California were obtained and individual images of the maxillary and mandibular models were produced using a video camera and an image capture card connected to a personal computer. According to the methodology employed, the author concluded that the golden ratio was found. In the relationship between the upper central incisor and lower central incisor in 25% of the material studied.

Amoric[4] reported in 1995 that the golden ratio has been studied by mathematicians and philosophers since antiquity, but it was the Renaissance artists who studied the golden number in greater depth. The author described that the golden ratio can be found in architectural constructions, in human beings and in nature. It can also be found in various cephalometric measurements and in various stages of craniofacial growth. In view of this, the author studied the possible golden ratio relationships between facial segments defined by cephalometric points in a sample aged between four and 18 years, using various tracings that are used by most professionals. A total of 19 tracings by different authors were grouped together to form this average figure. Using the golden compass, the author empirically listed the segments that could be in golden ratio. Once the reference numbers had been identified, he studied the variability of this proportion by accurately measuring the sizes of the facial structures and comparing them with the number 1.618 and multiples thereof. The author concluded that several craniofacial segments in golden ratio were found in many cephalometric measurements and at various stages of facial growth.

According to Jacobson[38] , 1995 in his book *Radiographic Cephalometry: from basics videoimaging* , treatment planning should seek to achieve the best aesthetics and function for each individual patient, rather than fitting them into the anatomical norms of ideal occlusion and the golden ratio of soft tissues and bone, can determine, at best, the best path for treatment planning; this should be done within an individual norm, derived from the specific characteristics of the patient analysed.

Zietsman *et al*.[116] (1995), reported that the golden ratio has been used by artists and architects to create their works. The application of the golden ratio to the human body is well documented by Lombardi[50] (1973) and

Levin[48] (1978). Ricketts[88] (1982) studied the golden ratio in lateral cephalometric radiographs. In view of this, the authors tested the measurements used by Ricketts[88] (1982) on the anterior face in a vertical plane and in a second proposal investigated the possibility of alternative points and proportions. The authors concluded that the segments studied are very close to the golden ratio and could be used in various areas of dentistry.

Mack[54] reported in 1996 that the lower third of the face has the greatest impact on the perception of facial aesthetics. An improvement in natural beauty can often be expected when accompanied by the restoration of the ideal relationship between dentition and facial soft tissue. The author reported that the golden ratio determined by the golden number 1.618 can be related to facial balance. It can be applied to determine the vertical dimension of occlusion and facial height, which the author considers to be the key to improving the beauty of the face. The author concluded that the goal of aesthetics should always be accompanied by the restoration of function.

Jefferson[40] (1996) reported on the golden ratio described by Ricketts[88] (1982). He also stated that the skeleton has a direct impact on facial appearance. Numerous articles in the literature have attempted to define facial beauty or aesthetics. Scholars have reported that facial beauty is subjective and culturally influenced. This type of thinking makes it impossible to establish a universal standard for the positioning of the skeleton. The author revealed that the golden ratio is directly related to facial beauty.

Suguino et al.[103] (1996), reported that the current concepts for diagnosis and treatment planning refer to the balance and harmony of facial features. Planning aesthetic facial changes is difficult, especially in terms of their integration with occlusion correction. Unfortunately, the treatment of malocclusion does not always lead to the correction or even maintenance of facial aesthetics. Sometimes, the enthusiasm to achieve a correct dental relationship can compromise facial balance. This can be partly due to a lack of understanding of what is desired as an aesthetic goal. The ability to recognise a beautiful face is innate, but translating it into objective and defined therapeutic goals becomes a more arduous task. The perception of beauty is an individual preference, with cultural influence. With the advance and popularity of orthognathic surgical procedures, the search for facial balance has become more prominent. This has intensified the need to study aesthetically balanced faces and the harmony between the different elements.

Zietsman *et al.*[115] , in 1997, proposed a list of points on the skull base where the maxilla could be positioned. The sample consisted of 100 lateral cephalometric radiographs. The authors concluded that the average distance between the glabella (Gl) and the phorium (Po) is in golden ratio to the average distance between the glabella (Gl) and point (A), and therefore the Po-glabella distance could be useful as a skull base reference for finding point (A), using the golden ratio.

In 1997, Garbin[27] used a sample of forty lateral cephalometric radiographs of forty young adults with normal dental occlusion. The author studied the relationship between the measurements of six Fibonacci golden ratios and a second objective was to assess whether the golden ratio manifested itself differently between individuals of different sexes. The author concluded that of the six ratios studied, five were in golden ratio for both males and females, and only one ratio was different between them.

Piccin[77] , also in 1997, checked the presence of the divine proportion by measuring photographs in a sample of 121 fully dentate young adult males and females. The subjects were positioned on a cephalostat, where they were photographed in the right lateral view, in the usual physiological resting position. The segments Lc-Sbn (corner of the eye to the base of the nose), Sbn-St (base of the nose to the stomium) and St-Gn (stomium to the extreme inferior and anterior point of the chin) were related. Using these segments as a basis, he analysed them statistically using the hypothesis test method and checked their correlation with the divine proportion, according to the ratio whereby the larger segment divided by the smaller segment equalled the sum of the two divided by the larger segment, resulting in the divine or golden number: 1.618. He concluded that there was a golden ratio between the Lc-Sbn and Sbn-St segments and between the Lc-Sbn and Sbn-Gn segments. Confirmation of these facial proportions in dentate individuals could help in oral rehabilitation and, more specifically, in obtaining the vertical dimension in totally or partially edentulous individuals who have a reduction in this dimension, and it could be checked whether these proportions were already present previously, using old photographs of these patients.

In 1998, Rufenacht[91] described ways of assessing facial morphology:

a) clinical, based on anatomical knowledge, which would be acquired through professional experience;

b) aesthetic, which would allow an appreciation of harmony and beauty, or by knowing or perceiving the aesthetic parameters that have been predetermined;

c) anthropometric, consisting of techniques for measuring the

body;

d) biometric, or a method that would use and exploit numerical factors.

Rufenacht also proposed dividing the face into three zones, called facial zones: the upper one, from the beginning of the forehead to the interpupillary line, related to cerebral activity, the middle one, which runs from the interpupillary line to the base of the nose and is related to social and sentimental activity, and the lower one, which runs from the base of the nose to the chin and is related to instinctive and psychic activity. Each of these parts is further subdivided into three others. The identical development of the three facial zones would lead to a psychomorphological balance and aesthetic harmony. When there is a predominance of one of the facial zones, aesthetic and morphological harmony will prevail, the balance will still exist, but it will emphasise the nature of dominance reflected by the facial composition.

Snow[98] (1999), reported that with the increased application of cosmetic dental treatment, a greater understanding of aesthetic principles has become necessary. Scientific analyses of the beautiful smile have repeatedly revealed objective principles that can be systematically applied to assess and improve dental aesthetics. Midline symmetry and regression following the golden ratio from anterior to posterior of the dental elements are required to create unity and an aesthetically pleasing smile. The golden ratio has been suggested as a possible mathematical tool for assessing the growth and proportion in the frontal norm of maxillary teeth, and the concept of the golden ratio has been proposed as a more useful application for assessing the aesthetics of anterior teeth.

In 1999, Garbin[28] checked the golden ratio in patients with Angle class III malocclusion, before and after orthognathic mandibular repositioning surgery, using a sample of twenty lateral cephalometric radiographs of ten young Brazilian leucodermic adults aged between 17 and 30 years, ten radiographs before and ten radiographs after orthognathic surgery. The author concluded that orthodontic-surgical treatment improved 97.76% of the proportions studied.

Eduardo[25] (2000) applied the golden ratio to guide the occlusal plan and re-establish the vertical dimension in edentulous individuals. The author pointed out that the loss of teeth leads to an aesthetic collapse of the patient, characterised by a more prognathic profile, a tendency for the lips and genital region to move into the oral cavity, leading to premature ageing. After observing the images of the lateral cephalometric radiographs of the patients assessed and carrying out a statistical analysis, he observed that the application of the divine proportion would be a reliable resource for determining the vertical dimension and providing facial harmony in edentulous patients, regardless of professional sensitivity. Of the eight measurements adopted in his methodology, two were more precise (Po - wing of the nose - inner corner of the eye and inner corner of the eye - wing of the nose - stomium), and the latter, as well as not depending on facial type, made it possible to check whether the upper plane of the face was within the correct limit.

Vegter & Hage[11] °(2000) carried out a research study in which they reviewed the literature on clinical anthropometry and facial aesthetics. The authors cited the importance of the golden ratio for Renaissance artists. The authors reported that the concepts of the golden ratio have been used to plan and evaluate treatments, especially in aesthetic plastic surgery, as a guide for correcting deformities.

Shinozaki[95] (2000) reported in his research paper on the unlimited capacity for aesthetic changes to the face due to the integration of orthodontic treatment, orthognathic surgery and plastic surgery, combined with facial orthopaedic techniques and knowledge of facial growth and development, indicating the need to develop systemic and consistent facial analyses. Attempts to predict the behaviour of soft tissue using measurements from cephalometric analyses of hard tissue often lead to aesthetic damage for the patient, making it necessary to study specific measurements for soft tissue and the behaviour of the facial profile. There is a need to use other branches of the sciences and the arts to define balanced aesthetics, as well as the use of various complementary analyses to obtain the correct development of the treatment plan with an emphasis on the soft tissue profile.

Baker & Woods[8] (2001), studied the changes in the number of facial proportions as a result of the combination of orthodontic treatment and orthognathic surgery. In the beautiful faces, the proportion values measured were close to the golden ratio (1.618:1). The authors stated that the changes in measurement values and consequently in facial proportions, as a result of combined orthognathic and orthodontic surgical treatment, would improve facial aesthetics. The authors used lateral and frontal cephalometric radiographs and pre- and post-treatment colour profile photographs of 46 patients, 36 of whom were women and ten men. Twenty-three of the patients underwent maxillary and mandibular surgery, four underwent maxillary surgery only and 19 underwent mandibular surgery. The photographs were assessed by 12 judges: two orthodontists, two oral and maxillofacial surgeons, two general dentists, two artists, two local people and two people involved in the fashion industry. Ten reasons that were in golden ratio in Ricketts' sample[88] (1982) were analysed in lateral cephalograms, pre- and post-treatment, and 11 reasons were analysed in frontal photos. However, the authors reported that there was no correlation between the aesthetic value and the golden ratio in the different faces, although the face proportions in some cases were in golden ratio after treatment. They concluded that if the golden ratio is to be used in the treatment plan for orthognathic surgery with combined orthodontic treatment, it should be in conjunction with other cephalometric analyses.

Araújo *et al.*[7] , in 2001 carried out a study analysing pre- and post-operative lateral cephalometric radiographs of the Fibonacci divine proportions described by Ricketts[88] (1982) in patients undergoing mandibular advancement. The sample consisted of ten leucoderma patients, regardless of gender, with ages ranging from 16 to 44 years. The patients had mandibular retrognathism with Angle Class II malocclusion and underwent surgery to correct it by sagittal osteotomy of the mandibular ramus. The authors concluded that in the sample used, "Fibonacci's divine proportions did not apply to the changes resulting from mandibular advancement surgery".

Gil & Mediei Filho[32] (2002), reported that there is a constant proportion that can be identified not only in the human body, but in nature in general. This constant is a proportion that seems to direct the growth, harmony, reproduction and stability of forms in nature. In this study, the authors assessed the craniofacial architecture of 23 adult males and females with normal occlusion, no previous orthodontic treatment and no tooth loss, using axial, frontal and lateral cephalometric radiographs. The search was carried out in the areas of force distribution and bone pillars, as well as in the areas of muscle insertions and natural divisions of the skull, as it is believed that proportion is a factor that directs balanced and harmonious growth and is more strongly related to the functions of the structures. The values of the selected measurements were obtained using the Radiocef programme from Radiomemory. The aim of this study was to verify the existence of the golden ratio in the cranial architecture of these individuals. Given the results obtained, the data was submitted to statistical analysis and the authors found 619 pairs of measurements in golden ratio, in at least 80% of the sample, 34 pairs in the axial incidence, 287 pairs in the frontal incidence and 298 in the lateral incidence. The authors concluded that the human skull has numerous golden ratio measurements in its structure, which interrelate in a variety of ways, giving it an efficient balance, suggesting that the skull, like other structures in nature, fulfils the requirements of the laws of energy conservation, tissue conservation and profound efficiency (Ricketts[88] ,1982).

Piselli[79] , 2003 evaluated the changes in a number of facial proportions as a result of orthodontic treatment using the golden ratio, and hypothesised that, as a result of orthodontic treatment, the vertical and horizontal dento-skeletal pattern of the patients in the sample would be more balanced and therefore the proportions measured after treatment should be closer to the golden ratio than before treatment. The sample used 36 lateral cephalometric radiographs taken before and after orthodontic treatment of 18 Brazilian female patients. All the patients had Class II malocclusion, 1° division. The authors concluded that of the four golden ratios evaluated, only one, Ena-Enp (p Enp-Mand, was found in the patients in the sample studied before and after orthodontic treatment; the Spog-A cp A-HF ratio was in the golden ratio at the start of treatment, but moved away from it at the end of orthodontic treatment. It is possible that patients with malocclusions do not have golden ratios, so if the golden ratio is used for orthodontic treatment planning in Class II, 1° division patients, it would be advisable to use it as an aid to other diagnostic methods.

Silva[96] (2003) evaluated how cephalometric measurements look in relation to the divine proportion, in a total of 52 proportions made up of 28 cephalometric points. He used lateral cephalometric radiographs of forty adult patients aged between 17 and 45, 13 males and 27 females, with Angle Class II malocclusion. The distances were measured using Radiocef Studio software. The data was submitted to statistical analysis and the author concluded that an average percentage of 65.48% of the cephalometric measurements were in golden ratio. The constitution of the skull architecture of the individuals influenced the variation in the percentage of divine proportions, because when relationships involved in areas of the skull more subject to variations due to malocclusion were used, there was a reduction in the percentage of golden proportions. The lower third of the head, together with the areas in the dental arches of the individuals in the sample, were the regions in which the proportions, among the cephalometric measurements studied, showed the lowest golden ratio percentages.

Marti ns[58] (2003) used lateral cephalometric radiographs to check for the presence of the golden ratio in segments of the craniofacial skeleton of individuals with normal occlusion who were at the peak of the pubertal growth spurt until before the end of skeletal maturation. The sample consisted of thirty lateral cephalometric radiographs and thirty hand and wrist radiographs obtained from thirty individuals with normal occlusion and without orthodontic treatment, aged between nine and 16 years, 17 females and 13 females. The sample was divided into two groups: group one included individuals who were at their peak two years later, while group two consisted of individuals who were between two and three years after their peak, but who had not yet reached skeletal maturity. The author concluded that there was no statistically significant difference in the number of golden ratios established by these segments between individuals who were in the peak pubertal growth spurt phase up to two to three years after the peak and before the end of skeletal maturation.

Araujo[6] (2003) analysed the occurrence of golden ratio

cephalometric measurements using lateral cephalometric radiographs in individuals on the ascending curve of the pubertal growth spurt who had normal occlusion and had not undergone previous orthodontic treatment. The study used 33 lateral cephalometric radiographs and 33 hand and wrist radiographs. They were aged between six and 13 years. For the cephalometric analysis, the author used part of the Lateral Golden Analysis created by Gil & Mediei Filho[32] (2002) in a programme called Radiocef, developed by Radiomemory. The sample was divided into three groups and the results were analysed statistically. The author concluded that there was no statistically significant difference in the quantitative values of the golden ratio between the three groups studied in the ascending curve of the pubertal growth spurt.

Santos[93] (2004) used 86 lateral cephalometric radiographs as a sample, which was subdivided into three groups according to the variation in the mandibular plane angle: G1 (24°>APM<27°), G2 (APM<24°) and G3 (APM>27°). In these groups, they observed the presence of the divine proportion, the facial proportions that could differentiate facial types, in the vertical direction and the spatial relationship of a rectangle with divine proportions, constructed in the lower third of the face with the Y ordinate. He found that in the three groups studied, the proportion of golden individuals was over 50%, groups G1, G2 and G3 and the facial proportion StGO': A'-B' were the elements capable of differentiating facial types in the vertical direction into mesofacial, brachyfacial and dolichofacial and that although the construction of the rectangle with divine proportions in the lower third of the face was possible in all the individuals in the sample, the manifestation of the positive golden ratio was only seen in groups G1 and G2.

Takeshita[104] (2004) checked the golden ratio on lateral cephalometric radiographs of 37 patients with Angle Class II malocclusion before and after orthodontic treatment. The author concluded that of the 19 ratios studied, eight differed in a statistically significant way, and seven of these eight were close to the golden number after treatment.

Walter-Porto[112] (2005) used lateral cephalometric radiographs of individuals aged between 17 and 25 years with Angle Class I malocclusion to check whether any measurements were in Golden Proportion in the craniofacial skeleton of 24 dolichofacial and 24 mesofacial individuals. Analysis of the results showed that, of the eight ratios studied, the Golden Ratio was present in four ratios in the group of mesofacial individuals and in only one ratio in the group of dolichofacial individuals.

Ono[72] (2005) checked whether certain ratios are in golden ratio in both brachyfacial and mesofacial individuals, and thus identified patterns that characterise these facial types, helping with treatment planning. Lateral cephalometric radiographs of 48 brachyfacial and 43 mesofacial individuals, aged between 17 and 25 years and with Angle Class I occlusion, were used. Of the eight ratios studied, four differed statistically between the two groups. The brachyfacial group did not present any of the ratios studied in golden ratio.

Castilho[2] °(2005) evaluated the golden ratio of skull and facial structures in individuals at the beginning and end of orthopaedic/orthodontic treatment. Ninety lateral cephalometric radiographs of 45 Brazilian leucodermic individuals treated orthopaedically and orthodontically were used. Two analyses were created based on the work of Gil & Mediei Filho[32] (2002), using the ratios that were in golden proportion by 80% and determining the importance of these ratios in treatment planning for the professional orthodontist and facial orthopedist. The author concluded that five ratios showed statistically significant differences in a favourable way, i.e. after treatment they moved closer to the golden number; 7 ratios did not show statistically significant differences and 3 ratios showed statistically significant differences in an unfavourable way, i.e. after treatment they moved away from the golden number.

Silva[97] (2005) evaluated the craniofacial golden ratio before and after orthodontic treatment, using photographs and lateral cephalometric radiographs. Forty-two adult subjects aged between 18 and 45 years were used, 21 males and 21 females, before and after orthodontic treatment using lateral cephalometric radiographs and lateral photographs. Of the four cephalometric ratios studied before and after orthodontic treatment, none had the average golden ratio. However, with orthodontic treatment, the average golden ratio was closer. Of the two photometric ratios assessed in this study, both were in divine proportion before and after orthodontic treatment, and one came even closer to divine proportion on average after treatment.

Martins[59] (2005) studied the proportions of equality and goldenness in craniofacial measurements using 59 lateral cephalometric radiographs obtained from individuals with normal occlusion who were in the growth period, 31 females and 28 males. The sample was subdivided into three groups (1, 2, 3) according to the Martins and Sakima growth curve programme (Radiomemory). Six ratios were used to assess the equality ratio and five ratios were selected to check the golden ratio. It was found that in group 1 the OPI-Pog/OPI-Ena ratio was in an equal proportion, but no golden ratio was found, in group 2 two ratios were statistically equal and two were in a golden ratio and in group 3 an equal proportion was observed in the N-Ena/Ena-Enp and ASPt-N/Ena-Enp ratios, while the presence of a golden ratio was only evident in the OPI-Enp/Ena-Enp ratio.

Dotto[24] (2006) analysed the golden ratio in lateral cephalometric measurements of individuals with Down syndrome (DS), as well as whether there were variations in the ratios assessed at different periods of growth according to the pubertal growth curve, and between male and female individuals. To this end, 52 lateral cephalometric radiographs and 52 hand and wrist radiographs of individuals with DS between six and 33 years of age were analysed. The sample was divided using the Growth Curve 1.0 programme (Radiomemory). 16 craniofacial segments were selected, generating 17 ratios. The results were analysed using Multiple Linear Regression and Student's T-test (5%). The author concluded that of the 17 ratios studied, nine showed no tendency towards the golden ratio at any stage of growth for either sex.

Jahanbin *et al.*[39] (2010) evaluated the changes in smile perception following the approximation of some smile components to the golden ratio, either orthodontically or surgically. To do this, they selected ten women aged between 20 and 25 with pleasant smiles and no obvious malocclusions to take part in this study. Five standard photographs were taken of each participant in a posed smile, and the most natural one was selected and digitised into black and white photos. Ten anthropometric landmarks were detected in each image and 10 ratios, including Labial inferioris (Li) / right cheilion (RCh) - right antegonion (RAgo), subnasal (Sn) -Li / left cheilion (LCh) - left antegonion (LAgo), RCh -Ago / labial superior (Ls) -Li, LCh-LAgo / Ls-Li, Ch-Ch / Ls-Li, stomium (St) -Sn / St-Li, the width of the maxillary central incisor / height of the maxillary central suffix, Ls- the right canine (RCus) / RCh- RCus, Ls-left canine (LCus) / LCh-LCus and LCus-RCus / Ch-Ch were measured in each image. The numerators or denominators of the ratios mentioned were then altered in a way that mentioned that the divine ratio (1 / 1.618) was approximated. All 110 photographs were evaluated by 40 judges in 2 sessions, using a visual analogue scale. The intraclass correlation coefficient was also calculated (single measure, 0.644; F = 26.27; P <0.001). The significance level for this study was P = 0.05. The tests used to analyse the data were the general linear model, the Friedman and Wilcoxon tests. It was found that bringing the RCus-LCus / Ch-Ch ratio closer to the divine proportion can definitely help achieve a more pleasing smile. At the next level, altering the Ls-LCus / LCh-LCus and Ls-RCus / RCh-RCus ratios could also play a role in making a beautiful smile.

Brum *et al.*™ (2010) analysed whether orthodontic treatment using the Ricketts Bioprogressive technique caused beneficial changes or not in the auric proportions assessed. To this end, 54 lateral cephalograms were taken before and after complete orthodontic treatment of a sample of 27 patients of both genders with Class II, division 1 malocclusion. They had a mean age of 10.5 and 16.5 years at the start and end of orthodontic treatment, respectively. The cephalometric assessment showed that the golden proportions (A-1/1-Pm; Xi-6/Xi-Pm and 6- 1/6-PTV) showed a significant difference between the pre- and post-treatment values and the proportions (FH-A/A-PM and Xi-Co/Xi-Pm) showed no significant change between the beginning and end of the orthodontic treatments carried out in this study. Four proportions (FH-A/A-Pm; A-1/1- Pm; Xi-6/Xi-Pm; and 6-1/6-PTV) were close to the golden value, while one (Xi-Co/Xi-Pm) was far from it. The third ratio (Xi-6/Xi-Pm) showed the best restoration compared to the golden value. Thus, they concluded that during the orthodontic treatment in question, most of the initial facial proportions that did not have values close to the divine proportion, came closer to the values considered ideal, with an aesthetic improvement of the face.

Packiriswamy *et al.*[73] (2012) studied facial morphology and identified 300 individuals with normal, short and long faces. The research participants were Malaysian nationals aged between 18 and 28 of Chinese, Indian and Malay extraction. The parameters measured were height and width of the face, and facial index was calculated. Face shape was categorised based on the golden ratio. Independent t-tests were used to test the difference between the sexes and between the races. The mean values of the measurements and the index showed significant sexual and interracial differences. Of the 300 individuals, the face shape was normal in 60 individuals, short in 224 individuals and long in 16 individuals. As anticipated, the measurements showed variations according to gender and race. Only 60 individuals had a regular face shape and the remaining 240 had an irregular face shape (short and long). As individuals with short and long shapes may be at risk of developing various disorders, knowledge of facial shapes in the given population is important for early diagnosis and treatment procedures.

Toniello *et al.*[106] (2014) investigated the golden ratio in lateral cephalometric radiographs of 93 Brazilian adults over 18 years of age, of both genders, with skeletal classes I, II and III, not undergoing orthodontic treatment, in lateral cephalometric radiographs, using the "Aurea Ceph" cephalometric *software*. Of the seven ratios studied, when the classes were evaluated, a statistically significant difference was found between the ratio (N-Ena/V1S-DM16) in classes I and III and the ratios (A-Pog/V1-C1MS and A-Pog/V1S-MD16) in classes II and III. When the ratios in the different classes were compared in relation to the golden number (1,618), there was a statistically significant difference in class I for the ratios (N-Ena/V1S-DM16, V1S-C1MS/C1MS-DM16 and Ena-Me/AB); in class II for the ratios (A-Pog/V1-C1MS and A-Pog/V1S-MD16); and in class III for the ratios (N-Ena/V1S-DM16, Ena-Enp/V1S-C1MS, V1S- C1MS/C1MS-DM16 and Ena-Me/AB).

Alam *et a/.*[1] (2015) investigated the association of facial proportion and its relationship to the golden ratio with the evaluation of facial appearance in the Malaysian population. This was a cross-sectional study of 286 randomly selected university students from University Sains Malaysia (USM) (150 females and 136 males; 100 Chinese Malays, 100 Malay Malays and 86 Indian Malays), with a mean age of 21.54 ± 1.56 (Age range, 18-25). The facial indices obtained from the direct facial measurements were used to classify facial shape into short, ideal and long. A validated structured questionnaire was used to assess the subjects' evaluation of their own facial appearance. The mean facial indices of Indian Malay (MI), Chinese Malay (MC) and Malay Malay (MM) were 1.59 ± 0.19, 1.57 ± 0.25 and 1.54 ± 0.23, respectively. Only MC showed significant sexual dimorphism in the facial index (P = 0.047; P <0.05), but there was no significant difference found between races. Of the 286 subjects, 49 (17.1%) were of ideal facial shape, 156 (54.5%) short and 81 (28.3%) long. The facial evaluation questionnaire showed that MC had the lowest satisfaction with a mean score of 2.18 ± 0.97 for the overall impression and 2.15 ± 1.04 for the facial parts, compared to MM and MI, with a mean of 1.80 ± 0.97 and 2.15 ± 1.04 for the facial parts.
1.64 ± 0.74 respectively for overall impression; 1.75 ± 0.95 and 1.70 ± 0.83

respectively for facial parts treatment. In conclusion: 1) Only 17.1 per cent of the Malaysian population's facial proportion conforms to the golden ratio, with the majority of the population having a short face (54.5 per cent); 2) facial indices do not depend significantly on race; 3) Significant sexual dimorphism was shown among Chinese Malays; 4) All three races are generally satisfied with their own facial appearance; 5) No significant association was found between the golden ratio and the facial evaluation score among the Malaysian population.In 2016, Bragatto *et al.*[5] analysed 110 lateral cephalometric tracings in the Dolping Imaging software, 55 before and 55 after orthognathic surgery, of patients with class II and III deformities and checked whether or not the 13 dentoskeletal indices, as defined by Ricketts, were close to the golden ratio. It was concluded that orthognathic surgery had little effect on the proportions studied, and that the golden ratio was not present in most of the indices analysed, either before or after surgery.

Walewski *et al.*[TM] (2017) verified the aesthetics of the facial profiles of Angle Class II and III patients before and after orthodontic-surgical treatment, as well as correlating 13 dentoskeletal ratios and five soft tissue ratios to the golden ratio. A total of 94 lateral cephalometric radiographs were analysed, in which 13 dentoskeletal ratios and five soft tissue ratios were measured and compared to the golden ratio. In addition, a subjective analysis of pre- and post-treatment facial aesthetics was carried out by 270 examiners. Dento-skeletal ratios 1, 3, 6, 7, 8 and 9 were close to the golden number after orthognathic surgery in Class III patients. For the soft profile, only ratio 4 came close to the golden number in both Class II and III patients. With regard to the subjective assessment of aesthetics, 91.49% of the facial profiles were considered more harmonious after treatment. It was concluded that, given the methodology used, the golden ratio has little influence on the assessment of facial aesthetics and does not serve as a guide for planning and orthosurgical treatment.

CHAPTER 5

Subjective assessment and photography in orthodontics

Stoner[102] , in 1955, carried out a study to provide evidence for assessing the profile of the lower third of the face. He collected 34 photographs of the faces of people he judged to have excellent harmony and beauty from orthodontic journals. He described the faces of these patients using angular measurements. He then selected 50 patients who had undergone orthodontic treatment in his private clinic. Observing the results of the photographic analysis of the pre- and post-treatment facial profile of the patients who underwent orthodontic treatment, he concluded that, for the patients considered to be balanced and possessing facial beauty, the angular values for the measurements that would describe the balance and beauty of the face were very close to the values previously calculated in his sample of 34 photographs of beautiful profiles.

Machado[53] (1974) emphasised that orthodontic diagnosis should not be a static procedure, but a continuous one, in order to be able to assess how far we have come and what needs to be done to achieve the proposed objectives and the best way to reach them. The author also reported that photography can be used to research and evaluate the progress of work, measure successes and recognise limitations. Therefore, he concluded that photography is an indispensable element in data collection, and for this it must follow certain technical standards in order to allow comparisons and study at any time, in a frontal or lateral view, serving as an element of study and discussion.

Claman *et al.*[21] (1990) reported that photography is becoming an increasingly important tool in dentistry. But documenting orthodontic or orthognathic treatment with pre- and post-treatment photographs can be misleading if the features in one or both photographs are distorted. The photographer must be constantly aware of the importance of standardising photographic variables and when the change in documentation is important. Although total reproducibility cannot be practised, the photographer can establish a reasonably standardised approach to photographing the patient.

In their work on facial aesthetics, Kerr & O'Donnell[42] (1990) reported on the attractiveness of photos of sixty patients, twenty of whom were in Class I, twenty in Class II Division 1 and twenty in Angle Class III. The photos were distributed to orthodontists, dental students, art students and the patients' parents. The authors concluded that art students and patients' parents were less critical in their assessment of facial attractiveness than orthodontists and dental students. In addition, the authors reported that the faces of patients with Angle Class II Division 1 and Angle Class III were less attractive than individuals with Class I occlusion.

In 1994, Michiels & Sather[62] evaluated the validity and agreement of the facial profile using vertical and horizontal dimensions on cephalometric radiographs and profile photographs. The aesthetic profile of 130 leucoderma women was assessed by 6 examiners. Vertical and horizontal assessments of the facial profile were made on cephalograms and profile photographs. A statistically significant difference was observed between the facial profile classifications in the photographs and lateral cephalometric radiographs. The authors concluded that the aesthetic objectives of orthodontic treatment should be based on facial changes observed clinically or through photographs.

Bishara *et al.*[13] (1995) used facial photographs of 91 patients to compare the changes in the soft tissue profile of people with Class II division 1 malocclusion who were treated with or without tooth extraction. The authors reported that:

> a) the photographs allow the profile structures to be measured;

b) in general, measurements from frontal photographs were more reliable than those obtained from lateral photographs and linear measurements were more reliable than angular ones.

Okuyama & Martins[70] (1997) researched the preference of the integumentary facial profile in young leucoderma, xanthoderma and melanoderma males and females, assessed by orthodontists, laypeople and plastic artists. The sample consisted of 180 photographs and the assessors categorised the profiles as good, fair and poor. Analysing the 21 preferred profiles, it was observed that all of them had a gentle facial convexity, greater for melanoderms and less for leucoderms; a greater nasal protrusion for males than for females; less lip convexity for female melanoderms compared to males and greater for female leucoderms than those of the opposite sex. The authors also reported that beauty can be defined as a state of harmony and balance of facial proportions, established by skeletal structures, teeth and soft tissues.

Bittencourt[14] (1999) stated that at the present time, it is not only desirable but essential to have complete and comprehensive documentation of the treatments carried out. The main aim of clinical photography is to record as much information as possible under reproducible conditions, and the application of photography in everyday activities should be a daily practice. Some professionals use photography simply as a means of recording and keeping a visual image of each treatment. Others want to have material that can be published or taught. Regardless of the objective, without the right knowledge and equipment, it is almost impossible to produce quality results.

Spyropulos & Halazonetis[101] (2001) reported that facial aesthetics is one of the main objectives of orthodontic treatment, and the emphasis placed on it has increased in recent years by patients and professionals when planning orthodontic treatment. Traditional orthodontics uses profile sketches to assess facial beauty. In the same vein, studies of facial aesthetics in orthodontic literature have concentrated on the facial profile aspect, especially the soft profile obtained from photographs or cephalometric radiographs.

Arguing that the vast majority of the population is in constant search of beauty, Landgraf et al.[45] (2002) showed that this demand for orthodontic treatment motivates professionals in the field of orthodontics and related disciplines to intensify their efforts, directing treatment planning towards the patient's aesthetic needs. They concluded that orthodontic diagnosis using frontal and lateral photographs complemented cephalometric analysis, satisfying patients' aesthetic desires and offering them a functional occlusion with the best possible results in terms of facial harmony.

Trevisan[108] (2003) reported in his research paper that facial profile analysis has long been of interest to orthodontic researchers, and several studies have been carried out to assess the facial profile in terms of its pleasantness or changes induced by orthodontic or ortho-surgical treatment. The author used profile photographs that were subjectively evaluated. Among the results obtained, it was found that natural normal occlusion was not indicative of facial profile beauty, as 28 per cent of the profiles assessed were classified as unpleasant. It was also noted that the numerical values found in his research were very close to the values suggested in the literature, indicating that cephalometric measurements, when used without the aid of subjective facial analysis, would not be sufficient to detect facial beauty.

Santos[92] (2003) assessed the presence and frequency of golden proportions on the faces of young, leucodermic Brazilians with normal occlusion according to the Andrews classification[5] (1972), without previous orthodontic treatment, using standardised photographs in the natural lateral and frontal head position. The sample consisted of 56 individuals, 21 males and 35 females aged between 12 and 21, with an average age of 16.1 years. After statistically analysing the results, a total of 276 pairs of golden ratio measurements were found. Only the 53 pairs of measurements that were in golden ratio with results above 60% were considered in this study: thirty pairs in horizontal measurements (frontal photographs), eight pairs in vertical measurements (lateral photographs) and 15 pairs in horizontal and vertical measurements (frontal and lateral photographs).

Machado & Souki[52] (2004) in their research paper Simplifying the acquisition and use of digital images - scanners and digital cameras, reported on the importance of digital photography in dentistry, helping communication between professionals, facilitating the preparation of orthodontic diagnoses, as well as illustrating scientific communications at conferences, courses and publications, making it an excellent teaching and research tool. The authors reported in their research paper that in order to print digital images obtained by digital cameras with photographic quality, a certain colour must be used. resolution consistent with the final size of the final print. As the image size used for most of our routine orthodontic needs generally does not exceed 10 x 15 cm, we suggest a resolution of 2048 x 1,536 pixels (3 megapixels).

Colombo et al.[22] (2004) proposed presenting a frontal facial analysis at rest and during smiling. The authors reported that the patient should be treated from an aesthetic point of view and not just from a cephalometric and functional point of view. Treatment should have an occlusal objective that matches facial aesthetics.

Oliveira Júnior[71] (2006) analysed the relationship between the various aesthetic rules described in reading and the perception of beauty, in order to obtain information for the correct aesthetic diagnosis of patients. To this end, he used sixty male and female volunteers aged between twenty and thirty years, of whom two photographs were taken (face and smile). These were initially paired, from one to sixty for faces and from 61 to 120 for smiles, and subjected to two aesthetic analyses as described below:

> a) perception of beauty: the 120 photographs were mixed and presented to twenty examiners who classified them, according to their criteria and personal tastes, as beautiful

or not beautiful;

b) sheets of tracing paper previously cut out were then attached to the photographs and the eight symmetry and proportionality standards were traced and measured: vertical golden ratio of the face, horizontal golden ratio of the face, interpupillary line, median line, incisal plane, golden ratio of anterior/upper teeth, smile line, interdental contact ratio.

He observed that volunteers classified as more beautiful confirmed the presence of aesthetic norms in 73.33 per cent of evaluations, while volunteers perceived as not beautiful confirmed the aesthetic rules in only 38.33 per cent of cases. The author concluded that the norms of proportional symmetry directly influence the perception of beauty, regardless of personal tastes; the perceptibly more beautiful volunteers had a correspondence with the aesthetic norms of 73.33%, while the non-beautiful ones had a confirmation rate of only 38.33%. The most influential norms in the perception of beauty were the horizontal golden ratio of the face and the smile line, with a frequency of 86.6%. Despite having the highest frequency of norms in volunteers considered beautiful (43.3%), the golden ratio of the teeth was present in only 13.3% of those considered not beautiful.

Scolozzi et al.[94] (2011) retrospectively investigated the accuracy and reliability of a skeletal cephalometric analysis based on the divine proportion (Sassouni analysis) in predicting "divinely proportioned" faces in the treatment of dentofacial deformities. Pre-operative and post-operative photographs of 50 patients were analysed and the following 5 proportions were measured: (1) TR-AL: AL-ME, (2) ME-AL: AL- LC, (3) LC-CH: CH- ME, (4) LC-AL: AL-CH, and (5) ME-CH: CH-AL (TR indicates triquetrum; AL, alar rim; ME, menton; LC, lateral corner; CH, cheilion). For each proportion, the treatment effect on the absolute difference between the proportions and the golden number (<D) (1.618) was analysed statistically. The analyses were adjusted

for gender, age, type of dentofacial deformity (anteroposterior and/or vertical) and surgical technique (surgery of 1 mandible vs 2 maxillas with or without a genioplasty). In all cases, the facial proportions analysed were not significantly altered by the surgical treatment, except for the ME-CH: CH-AL (lower third of the face) ratio, which was significantly moved to 1.618 (P <0.01). The present study demonstrated that (1) the divine facial proportion can be well approximated and predicted just by a specific cephalometric analysis in the lower third of the face and (2) parameters such as age, gender, type of dentofacial deformity, type of surgery and so on, could potentially and significantly influence the final results towards the divine proportion.

Nguyen *et al.*[68] (2016) assessed whether the frontal facial soft tissue proportions of Vietnamese women correspond to the golden ratio (GP). Sixty frontal facial photographs of Vietnamese female students aged 19 were selected. The selected participants had a symmetrical face, Class I occlusion, complete lip closure and no history of trauma or orthodontic treatment. The photographic record was set up with a white backdrop, fill light, a reflector, a Canon 650D camera and the participants were asked to sit in a standard position. The Trichion (TR), Temporal soft tissue (TS), left lateral corner (LC), lateral nasal (LN), Chilion (CH) and Menton (ME) points were used for photometric measurements in CorelDRAW Graphic X3 software. It was attested that soft tissue facial proportions of Vietnamese women did not correspond to GP. Changing the lower third can create harmonious vertical facial proportions.

CHAPTER 6

METHODOLOGY

This experiment began after the approval of the research project by the Research Ethics Committee for human studies, of the UNIVERSIDADE ESTADUAL PAULISTA, CÂMPUS DE SÃO JOSÉ DOS CAMPOS, FACULDADE DE ODONTOLOGIA, by means of certificate Protocol No. 046/2005-PH/CEP (Annex-A), mentioning that it was in accordance with ethical principles, according to guidelines and norms regulating research involving human beings, according to resolution No. 196/96 of the National Health Council.

1 Sample

The research that led to this book used lateral cephalometric radiographs, frontal and lateral photographs of 67 individuals aged between 12 and 27 years, obtained from the Radiology archive of the São José dos Campos Dental School (UNESP);

1.1 Sample selection

Lateral cephalometric radiographs and frontal and lateral photographs of adult males and females were selected.
of 67 female subjects totalling 134 lateral cephalometric radiographs, 134 frontal photographs and 134 lateral photographs:

> a) patients who have started and finished orthodontic treatment;
> b) patients without other craniofacial   deformities, syndromes or cleft palates.

2 Methods

2.1 The following methods were used:

> a) Adobe Photoshop 7.0 *for Windows* image manipulation software (Adobe Systems Corporation, USA);
>
> b) Excel XP *for Windows* statistical analysis software (Microsoft Corporation, Washington, USA);
>
> c) computer programme for statistical analysis, Minitab 13 *for Windows* (Minitab Inc, State College, USA);
>
> d) computer programme for statistical analysis, SPSS 11.0 *for Windows* (Lead Technologies, USA);
>
> e) Delphi 7.0 computer programme (Borland Software Corporation, USA);
>
> f) Aurea Ceph 3.0 computer programme for cephalometric analysis, specially developed for this research project;
>
> g) computer programme for viewing Photoview 2.0 images specially developed for
>
> visualisation of the photographic images in this research project;
>
> h) HP Compaq computer - AMD Turion 64 (HP, Washington, USA);
>
> i) HP Scanjet 4C scanner with adapter for transparency reader (HP, Washington, USA).

2. 2Development of a cephalometry programme.

For this research project, a cephalometry programme was created specifically to carry out cephalometric analysis, therefore not using the cephalometry programmes commonly found on the market. The programme was called Aurea Ceph, and its final version is currently 3.0, i.e. new versions have been devised, but the one that satisfactorily met the needs of this research project was version 3.0. The programming language used was Object Pascal using the Delphi 7.0 platform.

The programme was developed based on the cephalometric analysis created for this research project. The following algorithm was used to determine the distances between two randomly marked points:

$$a^2 = b^2 + c^2$$, which in programming language corresponds to:

```
procedure     TPlanilha.Button1Click(Sender:
TObject);
var a, b ,c
begin
a:=sqrt(b*b+c*c);
end
```

FIGURE 25 - Formula for calculating distances

2.3 Hardware and Software recommended requirements for using Aurea Ceph 3.0 (Computer and operating system).

a) Pentium III or higher microcomputer with 256 Mbytes of RAM;

b) monitor with a video configuration with a resolution of 1280X768 pixels and a screen size of 96 dpi (dots per inch);

c) recommended hard disc space: 10 Mbytes;

d) Windows XP or higher;

(e) desktop scanner, A4 size with adapter for transparency reader.

3 Radiographic analysis

a) the linear measurements were taken using the Aurea Ceph 3.0 programme (Figure 26). The Aurea Ceph 3.0 programme was developed in Delphi 7.0

(*Object Pascal* language*)*, especially for making cephalometric tracings, offers various features for better localisation of the cephalometric points, such as greater or lesser brightness, greater or lesser contrast, edge highlighting and zooming in on regions of interest. It is also possible to take measurements on photographs, as the programme has a calibration tool that generates a correction factor by simply entering a known distance on the image;

b) In this study, it was necessary to develop a new analysis for the radiographic study; new cephalometric points were created in the programme. The programme asks for a name for the point, an abbreviation and a definition of the anatomical location visualised on the screen. To check the golden ratio, we used the studies by Gil[25] (1999), Gil[26] (2001) and Gil & Mediei Filho[27] (2002). All the points, factors and ratios used by them served as a basis for this study (Figure 26 and Table 1);

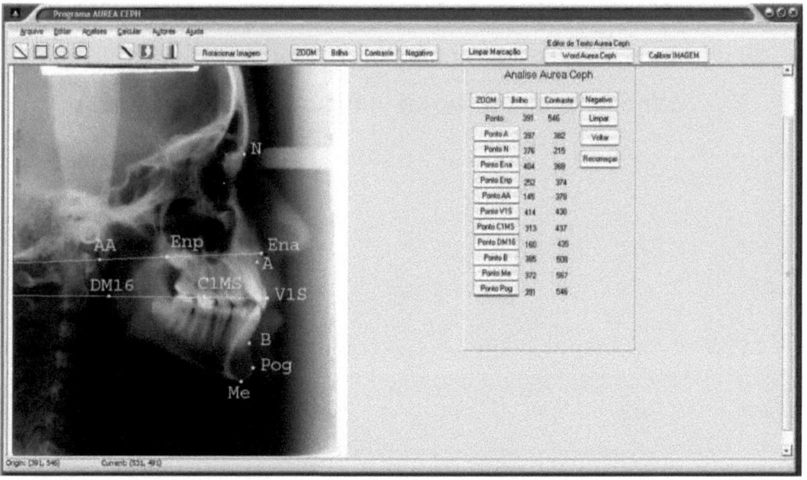

FIGURE 26 - Cephalometric points marked in the Aurea Ceph 3.0 programme.

Table 1 - Points used for lateral cephalometric analysis (continued)

N°	Abbreviation	Defining the point anatomically
1	A	Deepest point in the maxillary concavity between the anterior nasal spine and the alveolar ridge
2	N	Most anterior point of the fronto-nasal suture
3	Wow	Most anterior point of the maxilla
4	Enp	Most posterior point of the jaw
5	AA	Insertion of the extension of the maxillary plane with the posterior edge of the mandibular ramus
6	V1S	Point on the buccal side of the upper incisor, at C1MS height
7	C1MS	Point in the centre of the upper first molar
8	DM16	Point distal to the mandible, at the height of the C1MS-V1S line
9	B	Deepest point of the anterior concavity of the mandibular symphysis
11	Me	Lower point of the mandibular symphysis contour

c) after the markings have been made, the Aurea Ceph 3.0 software allows you to calculate the golden ratio by generating an Excel file, the values of which can then be analysed.

opened in the Excel XP programme, to determine the ratios to be used in this research study, we considered the work of Takeshita[95] (2004), which verified the golden ratio in patients before and after orthodontic treatment and also ratios considered important for professional orthodontists, as shown in Figure 27 and Table 2;

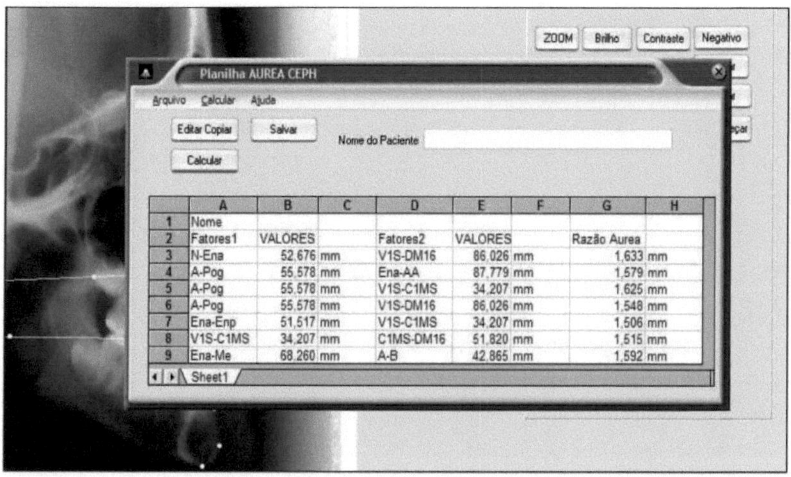

FIGURE 27 - Aurea Ceph 3.0 programme with the golden ratios used in the research.

Table 2 - The following reasons were used to carry out this work.

Patient's name:				
Factor 1	Values (mm)	Factor 2	Values (mm)	Reason value
N-Ena	0.000 mm	V1S-DM16	0.000 mm	0,000
A-Pog	0.000 mm	Ena-AA	0.000 mm	0,000
A-Pog	0.000 mm	V1S-C1MS	0.000 mm	0,000
A-Pog	0.000 mm	V1S-DM16	0.000 mm	0,000
Ena-Enp	0.000 mm	V1S-C1MS	0.000 mm	0,000
V1S-C1MS	0.000 mm	C1MS-DM16	0.000 mm	0,000
Wow me	0.000 mm	A-B	0.000 mm	0,000

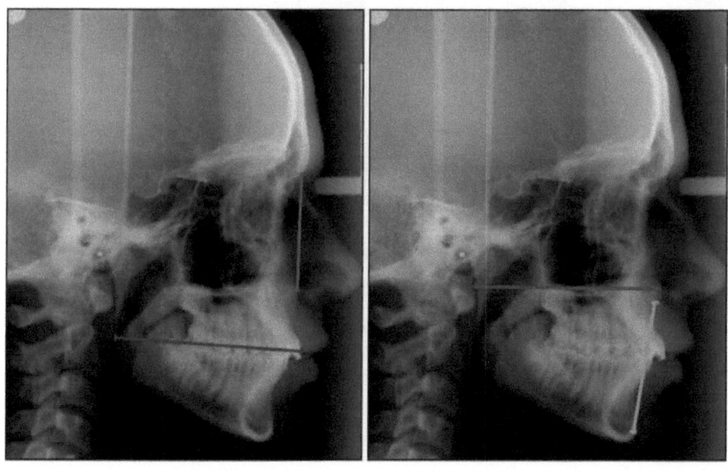

FIGURA 28   - Radiographic image of the N-Ena/V1S-DM16 and A-Pog/Ena-AA ratios.

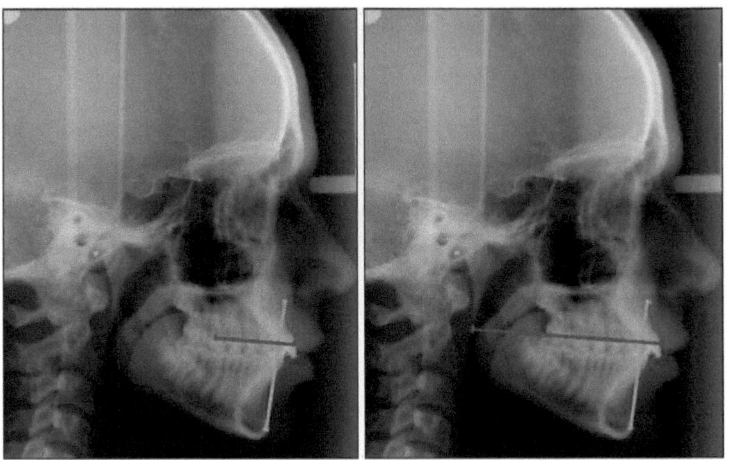

FIGURA 29   - Radiographic image of the A-Pog/V1S-C1MS and A-Pog/V1S-DM16 ratios.

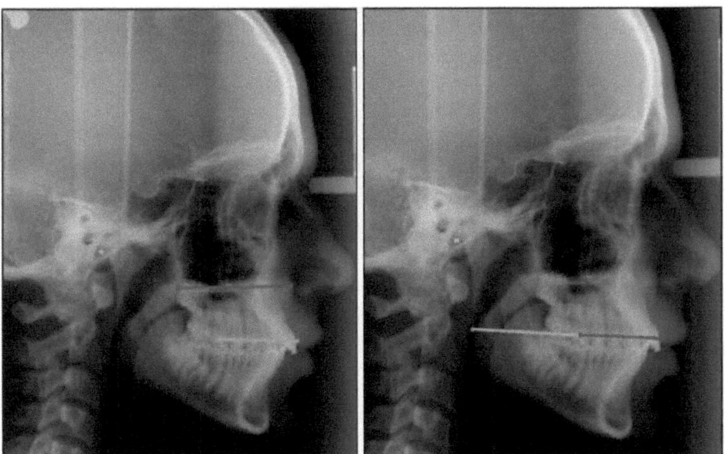

FIGURE 30 - X-ray image of the Ena-Enp/V1S-C1MS and V1S- C1MS/C1MS-DM16 ratios.

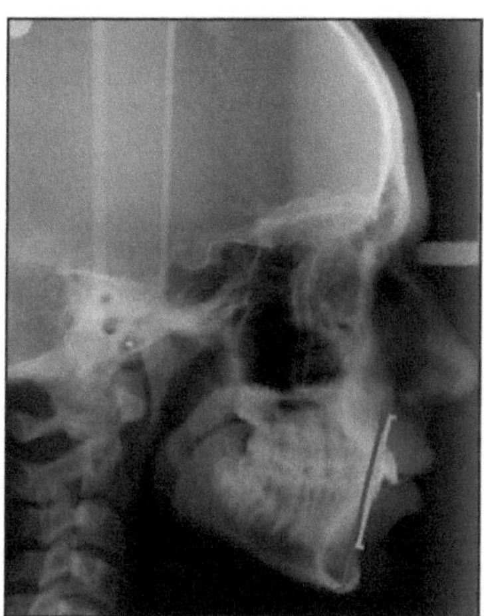

FIGURE 31 - Radiographic image of the Ena-Me/A-B ratio

4 Subjective evaluation of photographs

a) The photographs were scanned using an HP 4C *scanner* with a transparency reader (Hewellet Packward, Washington, USA), and then the images were recorded on a CD *(compact disk* - Sony, Oradell, USA) and inserted into Adobe Photoshop 7.0 to cut out the patients' faces and transform them into shades of grey;

b) In order to visualise the photographic images, a computer programme was developed on the Delphi 7.0 platform, called Photoview 2.0 (Figure 32). By clicking on the images, the programme generates a database, which can be saved in Excel file format, making it possible to carry out the statistical work. One thing to note is the reliability of exporting the data directly to the statistical programme without having to type in the data, which can lead to errors (Figure 33).

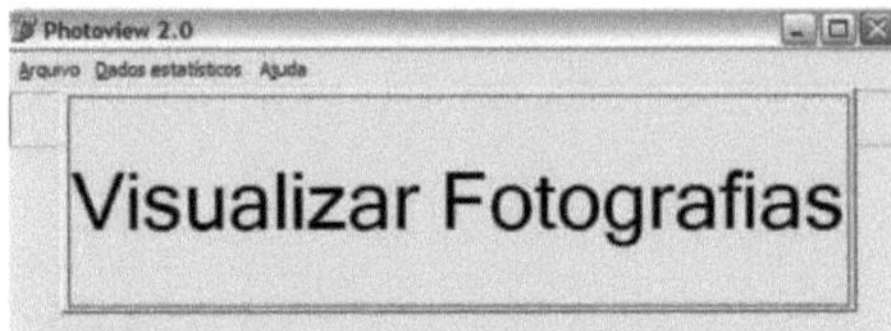

FIGURE 32 - Programme for viewing photographs.

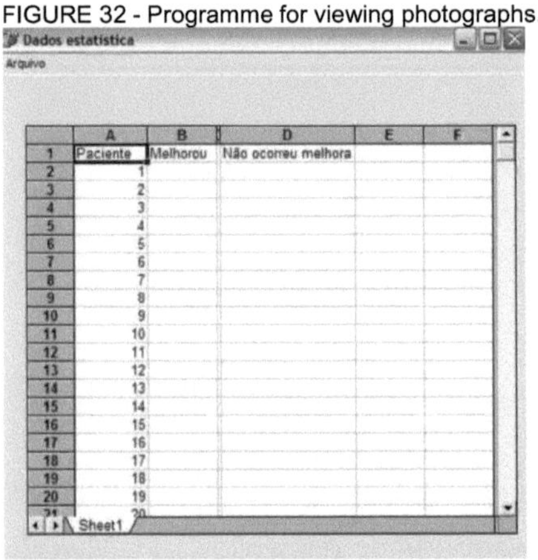

FIGURE 33 - Data exported directly into the statistical programme.

c) the frontal and lateral photographic images were evaluated before and after treatment by nine examiners, dental surgeons;

d) the examiners based themselves on two alternatives. There was an improvement in the aesthetics of the individuals compared before and after orthodontic treatment and there was no improvement in the aesthetics of the individuals compared before and after orthodontic treatment, by clicking on the buttons.

5 Statistical analysis

After the examiners had analysed the data and made the cephalometric tracings, they were compared and a statistical analysis was made of the relationship between the radiographic results obtained and the examiners' assessment.

examiners, thus verifying the relationship between facial aesthetics and the golden ratio in lateral cephalometric radiographs before and after orthodontic treatment.

Firstly, in order to divide the sample, the examiners made a subjective assessment of the photographic images, and the individuals were grouped into two groups:

    a) group 1 - aesthetic improvement compared before and after orthodontic treatment;

    b) group 2 - there was no aesthetic improvement when comparing before and after orthodontic treatment.

Once the ratio values were available, using the Minitab 13 *for Windows* software (Minitab Inc, State College, USA), the data was then submitted to descriptive statistical analysis (mean and standard deviation), using the paired t-test recommended by Baker & Woods[7] (2001), using a 95% confidence interval, in order to assess the behaviour of the ratios before and after orthodontic treatment.

The Student's t-test was then used to determine whether each ratio studied before and after orthodontic treatment could be considered golden. Applying this procedure, we verified the hypothesis that the average ratio of each golden group is 1.618. For this test we adopted a significance level of 5%.

To assess the presence of error in marking the cephalometric points and in the measurements taken in this research study, a second marking was carried out 15 days after the first marking. To assess the error, the analyses were submitted to linear regression analysis, which estimates the degree of agreement between two values obtained on different occasions. According to Houston[30] (1983), Martins et al.[51] (1995), Lofredo[43] (1996), Albuquerque & Almeida[1] (1998) and establishing the precision of the error involved is utopian and unrealistic, what should be done is to estimate the error.

CHAPTER 7

RESULTS

After obtaining the data, it was sent for statistical analysis. The results of this study will be presented in order to maintain the sequence of the procedures used to obtain the measurements.

1 Statistical analysis of the examiners' evaluation

The initial programme used was Microsoft Excel for Windows, version 2003 (Microsoft Corporation, Washington, USA). The division of the sample consisted of a subjective evaluation of the photographic images by the examiners, with the individuals being grouped into two groups:

a) group 1 - aesthetic improvement compared before and after orthodontic treatment;

b) group 2 - there was no aesthetic improvement when comparing before and after orthodontic treatment.

The subjective assessment used 67 individuals who had frontal and lateral photographs taken before and after orthodontic treatment. After the examiners had analysed the patients, they were subjected to the Z-test (Table 1).

Table - Statistical analysis of the examiners' subjective assessment (continued)

Patients	$Z(P = 0,5?)$-	$Z(p = 0.5?)$-	p-value =
Patient	0,888889	2,333333	0,009815*
Patient2	0	-3	0,00135*
Patient3	0,555556	0,333333	0,369441
Patient4	0,555556	0,333333	0,369441
Patient	0,222222	-1,66667	0,04779*
Patient6	0,222222	-1,66667	0,04779*
Patient?	0,888889	2,333333	0,009815*
Patient8	0,333333	-1	0,158655
Patient9	0,333333	-1	0,158655
Patienti 0	0,777778	1,666667	0,04779*
Patient 1	0,333333	-1	0,158655
Patient 2	0,333333	-1	0,158655
Patient13	0,222222	-1,66667	0,04779*
Patient 4	0,777778	1,666667	0,04779*
Patient15	0,777778	1,666667	0,04779*
Patient16	0	-3	0,00135*
Patient?	0,222222	-1,66667	0,04779*
Patient18	0,333333	-1	0,158655
Patient 9	0,111111	-2,33333	0,009815*
Patient20	0,111111	-2,33333	0,009815*
Patient21	0,777778	1,666667	0,04779*
Patient22	0,444444	-0,33333	0,369441

Patients	Zin = 0.5?) -	Z(p = 0.5?) -	p-value =
Patient23	0,444444	-0,33333	0,369441
Patient24	0,777778	1,666667	0,04779*
Patient25	0,444444	-0,33333	0,369441
Patient26	0,777778	1,666667	0,04779*
Patient27	0,222222	-1,66667	0,04779*
Patient28	0,222222	-1,66667	0,04779*
Patient29	0,444444	-0,33333	0,369441
Patient30	0,444444	-0,33333	0,369441
Patient31	0,333333	-1	0,158655
Patient32	0,777778	1,666667	0,04779*
Patient33	0,555556	0,333333	0,369441
Patient34	0,777778	1,666667	0,04779*
Patient35	0	-3	0,00135*
Patient36	0,222222	-1,66667	0,04779*
Patient37	0,222222	-1,66667	0,04779*
Patient38	0	-3	0,00135*
Patient39	0,888889	2,333333	0,009815*
Patient40	0,777778	1,666667	0,04779*
Patient41	0,777778	1,666667	0,04779*
Patient42	0,777778	1,666667	0,04779*
Patient43	0,444444	-0,33333	0,369441

Table 1 - Statistical analysis of the examiners' subjective assessment(conclusion)

Patients	Zin = 0.5?) -	Z(p = 0.5?) -	p-value =
Patient44	0,777778	1,666667	0,04779*
Patient45	0,777778	1,666667	0,04779*
Patient46	0,777778	1,666667	0,04779*
Patient47	0,333333	-1	0,158655
Patient48	0,777778	1,666667	0,04779*
Patient49	0,555556	0,333333	0,369441
Patient	0,111111	-2,33333	0,009815*
Patient51	0,777778	1,666667	0,04779*
Patient52	0,777778	1,666667	0,04779*
Patient53	0,777778	1,666667	0,04779*
Patient54	0,777778	1,666667	0,04779*
Patient	0,333333	-1	0,158655
Patient56	0,222222	-1,66667	0,04779*
Patient57	0,777778	1,666667	0,04779*
Patient58	0,444444	-0,33333	0,369441
Patient59	0	-3	0,00135*
Patient60	0,777778	1,666667	0,04779*
Patient61	0,222222	-1,66667	0,04779*
Patient62	0,444444	-0,33333	0,369441
Patient63	0,222222	-1,66667	0,04779*
Patient64	0,888889	2,333333	0,009815*
Patient65	0,222222	-1,66667	0,04779*
Patient66	0,111111	-2,33333	0,009815*
Patient67	0,222222	-1,66667	0,04779*

'statistically significant difference at the 5% level

Individuals with results that differed statistically significantly at the 5% level were classified, those that did not differ statistically significantly at the 5% level, and there was no agreement between the examiners according to the test and degree of significance used, so this group of a total of twenty patients were excluded from the total sample, thus establishing 47 individuals who were divided into 2 groups:

a) Group 1 - Aesthetic improvement compared before and

after orthodontic treatment;

b) group 2 - there was no aesthetic improvement when comparing before and after orthodontic treatment.

Distribuição dos pacientes pelos Examinadores

22 Pacientes

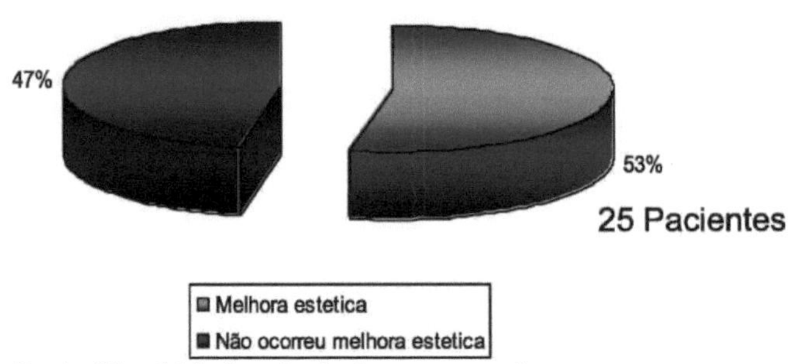

FIGURE 35 - Graph of the distribution of patients among examiners

2 Statistical analysis of the aesthetic improvement group

After dividing the sample, statistics were carried out for group 1 - Aesthetic improvement compared before and after orthodontic treatment. Fifty radiographs were used, 25 before and 25 after orthodontic treatment. Once the ratios had been obtained, the values were then submitted to statistical analysis. Using the paired "T" test, it is possible to calculate the mean of the ratios of the 25 patients and the standard deviation, using the 95% Confidence Interval, thus observing the statistical behaviour of the ratios studied in this research study. However, before assessing the statistical behaviour of the ratios, the intra-examiner error was assessed. The 11 points were marked twice on each lateral cephalometric radiograph, considering a 30-day interval between the markings. These markings were made by a single previously trained examiner. The 11 anatomical points generated nine factors, with each factor representing a cranial measurement in millimetres. The measurements obtained at the two different times (initial and thirty days later) were subjected to linear regression analysis, which checked for the presence of casual and systematic measurement errors.

Table 2 - Results corresponding to the intra-examiner error values for each factor in the 47 individuals.

Factors	Value of r
N-Ena	0,986
A-Pog	0,973
Ena-Enp	0,979
V1S-C1MS	0,967
Wow me	0,969
V1S-DM16	0,984
Ena-AA	0,992
C1MS-DM16	0.968
A-B	0,951

Table 2 shows the values corresponding to the intra-examiner error obtained using the Linear Regression Analysis test between the factors. It can be seen that the correlation values (r) for the nine factors in this study were greater than 0.90, indicating a high correlation between the measurements at the two different times, so the measurements can be used to calculate the ratios in the study. Statistical analysis was then carried out.

2.1 Ratio   N-EnaA/1S-DM16

Table 3 - Paired T-Test (N-Ena/V1S-DM16)

Paired T-test R1 initial - R1 final			
X-rays	N	Average	Standard Deviation
Initial R1	25	1,61748	0,14144
R1 final	25	1,64116	0,08837
Difference	25	-0,023680	0,100037

95% confidence interval mean difference: (-0.064973; 0.017613)

p-value = 0.248 p>0.05 therefore not statistically different

2.   2A-Pog/Ena-AA ratio

Table 4 - Paired T-test (A-Pog/Ena-AA)

Paired T-test R1 initial - R1 final			
X-rays	N	Average	Standard Deviation
Initial R2	25	1,51772	0,16253
R2 final	25	1,48612	0,13056
Difference	25	0,031600	0,094091

95% confidence interval mean difference: (-0.007239; 0.070439)

p-value = 0.106 p>0.05 therefore not statistically different

2.3 Ratio   A-Pog/V1S-C1MS

Table 5 - Paired T-Test (A-Pog/V1S-C1 MS)

| Paired T-test R1 initial - R1 final | | | |
X-rays	N	Average	Standard Deviation
Initial R3	25	1,54196	0,19778
Final R3	25	1,68728	0,12876
Difference	25	-0,145320	0,155431

95% confidence interval mean difference: (-0.209479; -0.081161)

p-value = 0.000 p<0.05 therefore statistically different

2.4 Ratio   A-Pog/V1S-DM16

Table 6 - Paired T-Test (A-Pog/ V1S-DM16)

| Paired T-test R1 initial - R1 final | | | |
X-rays	N	Average	Standard Deviation
Initial R4	25	1,52712	0,18478
R4 final	25	1,55140	0,12061
Difference	25	-0,024280	0,130199

95% confidence interval mean difference: (-0.078024; 0.029464)

p-value = 0.360 p>0.05 therefore not statistically different

2.   5 Ena-Enp/V1S-C1MS ratio

Table 7 - Paired T-Test (Ena-Enp/V1S-C1MS)

| Paired T-test R1 initial - R1 final | | | |
X-rays	N	Average	Standard Deviation
Initial R5	25	1,38312	0,13569
R5 final	25	1,50828	0,08641
Difference	25	-0,125160	0,123654

95% confidence interval mean difference: (-0.176202; -0.074118)

p-value = 0.000 p<0.05 therefore statistically different

2.6 Ratio   V1S-C1MS/C1MS-DM16

Table 8 - Paired T-Test (V1S-C1MS/C1MS-DM16)

| Paired T-test R1 initial - R1 final | | | |
X-rays	N	Average	Standard Deviation
Initial R6	25	1,32700	0,20141
R6 final	25	1,60364	0,06539
Difference	25	-0,276640	0,193988

95% confidence interval mean difference: (-0.356714; -0.196566)

p-value = 0.000 p<0.05 therefore statistically different

2.7 Ena-Me/A-B ratio

Table 9 - Paired T-Test (Ena-Me/A-B)

| Paired T-test R1 initial - R1 final | | | |
X-rays	N	Average	Standard Deviation
Initial R7	25	1,62232	0,09701
R7 final	25	1,59940	0,07161

Difference	25	0,022920	0,096408

95% confidence interval mean difference: (-0.016875; 0.062715)

p-value = 0.246 p>0.05 therefore not statistically different

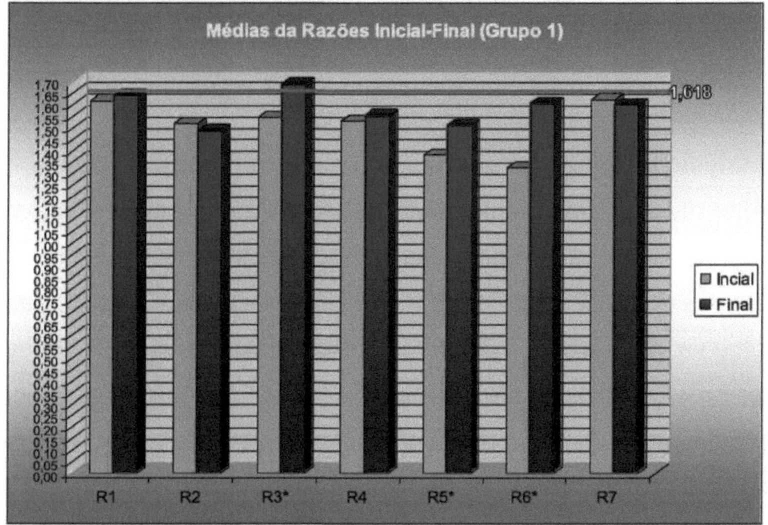

* statistically significant difference at 5% level

FIGURE 36 - Graph of the means of the initial-final ratios (Groupol)

In order to check whether the ratio studied could represent the golden number, Student's t-test was applied, with a 5% significance level. Using this test, each ratio before and after orthodontic treatment was compared to 1.618. The ratios studied, which could represent the golden number, were not statistically different from the golden number, i.e. the ratio that according to the statistics used is in golden proportion. When there is a statistically significant difference at the 5% level, it means that the ratio studied is not a golden ratio (Table 10).

Table 10 - Student's t-test results for the ratios studied

Reasons	N	Average	Standard Deviation	Range 95% confidence	T	P value
Initial R1	25	1,61748	0,14144	(1,55910; 1,67586)	-0,02	0,985
R1 final	25	1,64116	0,08837	(1,60468; 1,67764)	1,31	0,202
Initial R2	25	1,51772	0,16253	(1,45063; 1,58481)	-3,08	0,005*
R2 final	25	1,48612	0,13056	(1,43223; 1,54001)	-5,05	0,000*
Initial R3	25	1,54196	0,19778	(1,46032; 1,62360)	-1,92	0,067
Final R3	25	1,68728	0,12876	(1,63413; 1,74043)	2,69	0,013*
Initial R4	25	1,52712	0,18478	(1,45085; 1,60339)	-2,46	0,022*
R4 final	25	1,5514	0,12061	(1,50162; 1,60118)	-2,76	0,011*

Initial R5	25	1,38312	0,13569	(1,32711; 1,43913)	-8,66	0,000*
R5 final	25	1,50828	0,08641	(1,47261; 1,54395)	-6,35	0,000*
Initial R6	25	1,327	0,20141	(1,24386; 1,41014)	-7,22	0,000*
R6 final	25	1,60364	0,06539	(1,57665; 1,63063)	-1,1	0,283
Initial R7	25	1,62232	0,09701	(1,58227; 1,66237)	0,22	0,826
R7 final	25	1,5994	0,07161	(1,56984; 1,62896)	-1,3	0,206

'statistically significant difference at the 5% level

3 Statistical analysis of the group showed no aesthetic improvement

After dividing the sample, statistics were carried out for group 2 - No aesthetic improvement before and after orthodontic treatment - using 44 radiographs, 22 before and 22 after orthodontic treatment. Once the ratios had been obtained, the values were then submitted to statistical analysis. Using the paired t-test, it is possible to calculate the mean of the ratios of the 25 patients and the standard deviation. A 95% confidence interval was used to determine the statistical behaviour of the ratios studied in this study.

3.1 N-Ena/V1S-DM16 ratio

Table 11 - Paired T-Test (N-Ena/V1S-DM16)

Paired T-test R1 initial - R1 final			
X-rays	N	Average	Standard Deviation
Initial R1	22	1,63059	0,13908
R1 final	22	1,58364	0,12881
Difference	22	0,046955	0,076820

95% confidence interval mean difference: (0.012894; 0.081015)

p-value = 0.009 p<0.05 therefore statistically different

3.   2A-Pog/Ena-AA ratio

Table 12 - Paired T-test (A-Pog/Ena-AA)

Paired T-test R1 initial - R1 final			
X-rays	N	Average	Standard Deviation
Initial R2	22	1,50273	0,17524
R2 final	22	1,48114	0,15235
Difference	22	0,021591	0,094510

95% confidence interval mean difference: (-0.020312; 0.063494)

p-value = 0.296 p>0.05 therefore not statistically different

3.3Ratio   A-Pog/V1S-C1MS

Table 13 - Paired T-Test (A-Pog/V1 S-C1 MS)

| Paired T-test R1 initial - R1 final | | | |
X-rays	N	Average	Standard Deviation
Initial R3	22	1,51064	0,18224
Final R3	22	1,52918	0,17740
Difference	22	-0,018545	0,147765

95% confidence interval mean difference: (-0.084061; 0.046970)

p-value = 0.562 p>0.05 therefore not statistically different

3.4 Ratio   A-Pog/V1S-DM16

Table 14 - Paired T-Test (A-Pog/ V1S-DM16)

| Paired T-test R1 initial - R1 final | | | |
X-rays	N	Average	Standard Deviation
Initial R4	22	1,55423	0,15714
R4 final	22	1,52214	0,12014
Difference	22	0,032091	0,084927

95% confidence interval mean difference: (-0.005564; 0.069745)

p-value =0.091 p>0.05 therefore not statistically different

3.   5 Ena-Enp/V1S-C1MS ratio

Table 15 - Paired T-Test (Ena-Enp/V1S-C1 MS)

| Paired T-test R1 initial - R1 final | | | |
X-rays	N	Average	Standard Deviation
Initial R5	22	1,33059	0,14669
R5 final	22	1,37664	0,17019
Difference	22	-0,046045	0,127034

95% confidence interval mean difference: (-0.102369; 0.010278)

p-value = 0.104 p>0.05 therefore not statistically different

3.6 Ratio   V1S-C1MS/C1MS-DM16

Table 16 - Paired T-Test (V1S-C1MS/C1MS-DM16)

| Paired T-test R1 initial - R1 final | | | |
X-rays	N	Average	Standard Deviation
Initial R6	22	1,34691	0,21080
R6 final	22	1,30595	0,22124
Difference	22	0,040955	0,154022

95% confidence interval mean difference: (-0.027335; 0.109244)

p-value = 0.226 p>0.05 therefore not statistically different

3.7 Ena-Me/A-B ratio

Table 17 - Paired T-Test (Ena-Me/A-B)

Paired T-test R1 initial - R1 final

X-rays	N	Average	Standard Deviation
Initial R7	22	1,56232	0,09057
R7 final	22	1,58145	0,09705
Difference	22	-0,019136	0,106661

95% confidence interval mean difference: (-0.066427; 0.028154)

p-value = 0.410 p>0.05 therefore not statistically different

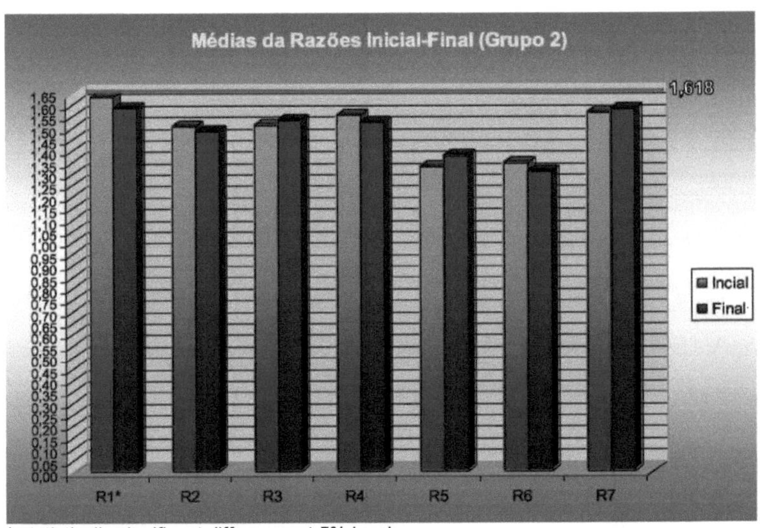

* statistically significant difference at 5% level

FIGURE 37 - Graph of the means of the initial-final ratios (Group 2)

In order to check whether the ratio studied could represent the golden number, Student's t-test was applied, with a 5% significance level. Using this test, each ratio before and after orthodontic treatment was compared to 1.618. Table 18.

Table 18 - Student's t-test results for the ratios studied (continued)

Reasons	N	Average	Standard Deviation	Range 95% confidence	T	value ofP
Initial R1	22	1,63059	0,13908	(1,56892; 1,69226)	0,42	0,675
R1 final	22	1,58364	0,12881	(1,52653; 1,64075)	-1,25	0,225
Initial R2	22	1,50273	0,17524	(1,42503; 1,58043)	-3,09	0,006*
R2 final	22	1,48114	0,15235	(1,41359; 1,54869)	-4,21	0,000*
Initial R3	22	1,51064	0,18224	(1,42983; 1,59144)	-2,76	0,012*
Final R3	22	1,52918	0,1774	(1,45053; 1,60784)	-2,35	0,029*

Initial R4	22	1,55423	0,15714	(1,48456; 1,62390)	-1,9	0,071
R4 final	22	1,52214	0,12014	(1,46887; 1,57540)	-3,74	0,001*
Initial R5	22	1,33059	0,14669	(1,26555; 1,39563)	-9,19	0,000*
R5 final	22	1,37664	0,17019	(1,30118; 1,45209)	-6,65	0,000*
Initial R6	22	1,34691	0,2108	(1,25345; 1,44037)	-6,03	0,000*
R6 final	22	1,30595	0,22124	(1,20786; 1,40405)	-6,62	0,000*
Initial R7	22	1,56232	0,09057	(1,52216; 1,60248)	-2,88	0,009*
R7 final	22	1,58145	0,09705	(1,53842; 1,62449)	-1,77	0,092

* statistically significant difference at 5% level

CHAPTER 8

DISCUSSION

The golden ratio has been known since ancient times and has been widely used in architecture and art, having been studied and described by many artists, philosophers and mathematicians. It can be observed in nature, for example in the distribution of petals in flowers, in the reproduction of animals, in the shape of animals and in human beings, and is the subject of study, especially in terms of its relationship with aesthetics [30].

Believing that the most stable, aesthetically pleasing, balanced and functionally efficient structures are in the golden ratio, and that the human skull, which fits these qualifications perfectly, should also be in the golden ratio, authors such as [29, 47, 86, 87, 88, 106, 107] decided to study it in dentistry and found this relationship in craniofacial measurements. These findings fuelled the development of many studies related to the golden ratio in dentistry.

The aim of the researchers was to create an individualised cephalometric analysis, i.e. far removed from the average standards of the population [4, 27, 30, 88]. This provides a further tool for professional dentists to seek facial harmony and aesthetics, and in the future, as studies progress, to use the golden ratio as an auxiliary method in treatment planning.

As well as restoring stable occlusion and improving function, dental professionals should also aim to improve and provide balance, harmony and facial aesthetics [10, 23, 30, 32, 39, 54, 85, 103, 109, 114].

Regarding the relationship between the golden ratio and facial aesthetics [4, 27, 29, 30, 31, 32, 39, 40, 71, 87, 88, 116], the authors revealed the presence of a relationship between the golden ratio and facial aesthetics. However, few authors have related the golden ratio and facial aesthetics before and after orthodontic treatment [15]. Trevisan (2003) [108] also observed that natural normal occlusion was not indicative of a beautiful facial profile. The numerical values found were very close to those suggested in the literature, indicating that cephalometric measurements, when used without the aid of subjective facial analysis, were not sufficient to detect facial beauty.

To obtain the distance between the segments, we used cephalometric points and factors measured from lateral cephalometric radiographs. To do this, we used the Aurea Ceph computer programme, which was developed in the Pascal language on the Delphi platform. The programme allows the ratios to be calculated directly, generating a report that can be saved in Excel file format, making it possible to carry out statistical work. One thing to note is the reliability of exporting the data directly to the statistical programme without the need to type in the data, which can lead to errors. According to Halazonetis (1994) [34], Martins *et al.* (1995) [57], Albuquerque & Almeida (1998) [2], Brangeli *et al.* (2000) [16] and Miquilito (2003) [63], Bragatto *et al* (2016) [15] reported that the indirect computerised method, using digitised images, when compared to the manual method, proved to be more reliable and have good reproducibility.

With regard to the statistical analysis of the subjective analysis, the sample consisted of photographs of 67 individuals before and after treatment. The subjects were assessed according to their aesthetic improvement compared before and after orthodontic treatment or not compared before and after orthodontic treatment. Individuals whose results showed a statistically significant difference at the 5% level were used, those who did not differ statistically significantly at the 5% level and there was no agreement between the examiners according to the Z-test and the degree of significance, were eliminated, from this group a total of twenty individuals were excluded from the sample, thus establishing 47 individuals who were divided into two groups: a) Aesthetic improvement compared before and after orthodontic treatment a total of 25 individuals and b) No aesthetic improvement compared before and after orthodontic treatment a total of 22 individuals (Figure 35).The results of the seven proportionality ratios used in this study are analysed below.

Ratio 1 (N-EnaA/1S-DM16) (Figure 38) relates a vertical segment in the middle third (N-Ena) and a horizontal segment (V1S- DM16), consisting of a point in the V1S dental region and another point in the distal mandible, at the height of the C1MS-V1S line.

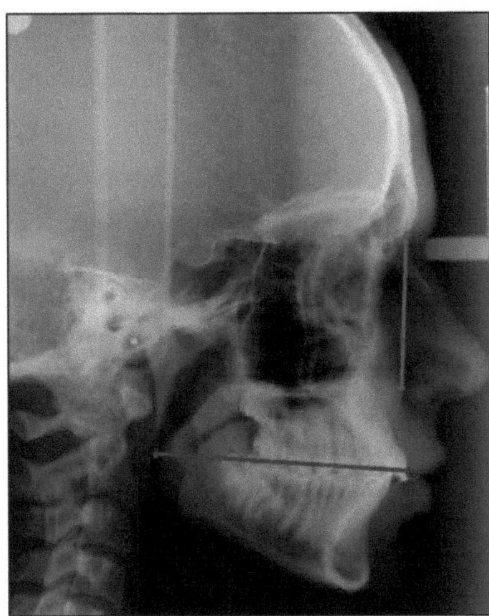

FIGURE 38 - Representative X-ray of the N-Er /V1S-DM16 ratio

In group 1, aesthetic improvement compared before and after orthodontic treatment, ratio 1, applying the paired t-test before and after orthodontic treatment, did not show a statistically significant difference and in the graph (Figure 36) the ratio compared before and after orthodontic treatment was closer on average to the golden number after orthodontic treatment [18]. In group 2, there was a statistically significant difference and there was also a distancing on average from the golden number compared before and after orthodontic treatment (Figure 37). However, in both groups, in order to check whether the ratio studied could statistically represent the golden number, Student's t-test was applied, adopting a 5% significance level; before treatment the ratio was in a golden proportion and after treatment it remained in a golden proportion. This was also observed by Gil (1999) [30], who found that the ratio was golden, although the sample consisted of individuals without orthodontic treatment and with normal occlusion.

In the research study by Takeshita (2004) [104], the ratio differed in a statistically significant way before and after orthodontic treatment, using the paired t-test, and there was an average approximation towards the golden number; however, the author used patients with Class II malocclusion as a sample. This ratio relates a vertical segment (N-Ena) at cephalometric points little influenced by treatment and another segment (V1S-DM16), as it is a horizontal distance in the region of the teeth that the orthodontist can modify with treatment [37].With regard to **ratio 2** (A-Pog/Ena-AA) (Figure 39), it relates a vertical segment between maxilla and mandible (A-Pog) and a horizontal segment (Ena-AA).

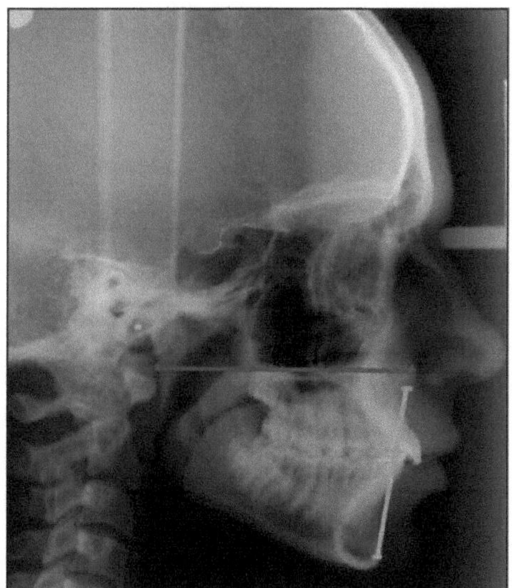

FIGURE 39 - Representative X-ray of the Ena-AA ratio

Both groups 1 and 2 did not differ statistically significantly in the paired t-test at the 5% level, compared before and after orthodontic treatment. Applying the t-test at the

5% significance level in order to verify the presence of the golden ratio in both groups were outside the golden ratio before orthodontic treatment and continued to be outside after orthodontic treatment. In the graphs (Figures 36 and 37), in groups 1 and 2 we can see that the results were on average far from the golden number. This may have occurred due to the stability of the cephalometric points in this region, when related to the Ena-AA segment, and the difficulty of altering the vertical A-pog distances [37]. Furthermore, in the case of the A-Pog segment, it is modified by mandibular growth [83], which is independent of the orthodontist's actions.

Ratio 3 (A-Pog/V1S-C1MS) (Figure 40) relates a vertical segment between the maxilla and mandible (A-Pog) and a horizontal segment formed with cephalometric points on teeth (V1S-C1MS).

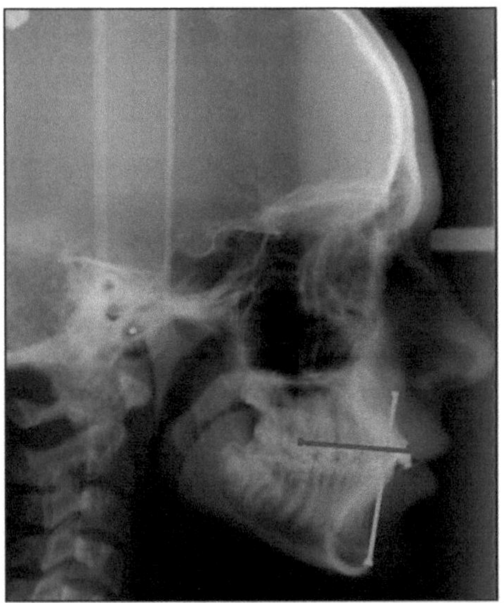

FIGURE 40 - Representative X-ray of the A-P< V1S-C1MS ratio

Group 1 showed a statistically significant difference when compared before and after orthodontic treatment. The graph (Figure 36) comparing before and after orthodontic treatment shows an approximation to the golden number after orthodontic treatment. In group 2 there was no statistically significant difference, but the graph (Figure 37) shows a slight approximation in relation to the golden number. Applying the t-test at the 5% significance level in order to verify the presence of a golden ratio, group 1 was in a golden ratio before treatment and after treatment it was no longer in a golden ratio; in group 2, both before and after, the ratio was in a golden ratio.

Ratio 4 (A-Pog/ V1S-DM16) (Figure 41) relates a vertical segment between the maxilla and mandible (A-Pog) and a horizontal segment (V1S-DM16), consisting of a point in the V1S dental region and another point distal to the mandible, at the C1MS-V1S line.

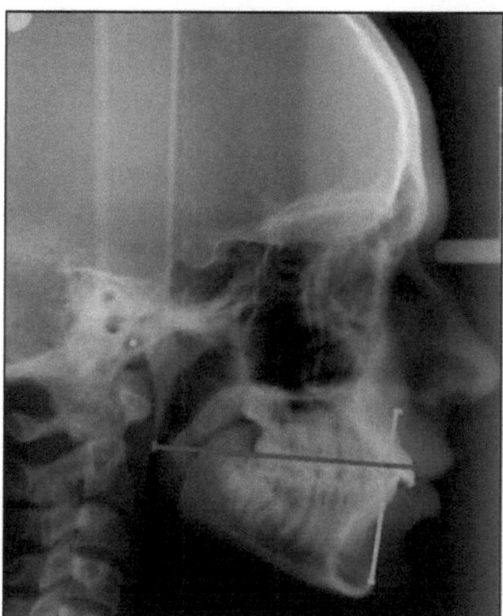

FIGURE 41 - Representative X-ray of the V1S-DM16 A-Pi ratio

In group 1 and 2 there was no statistically significant difference compared to the paired t-test. The graph (Figure 36), which represents group 1, shows an average approximation to the golden number. However, when compared to the graph (Figure 37), which corresponds to group 2, there is a distance from the golden number. Applying the t-test at the 5% significance level in order to verify the presence of the golden ratio, group 1 before and after orthodontic treatment were not in the golden ratio, group 2 before was in the golden ratio and after treatment was no longer in the golden ratio.

Ratio 5 (Ena-Enp/V1S-C1MS) (Figure 42) relates two horizontal segments, one in the maxilla (Ena-Enp) and the other in the maxilla in teeth (V1S-DM16).

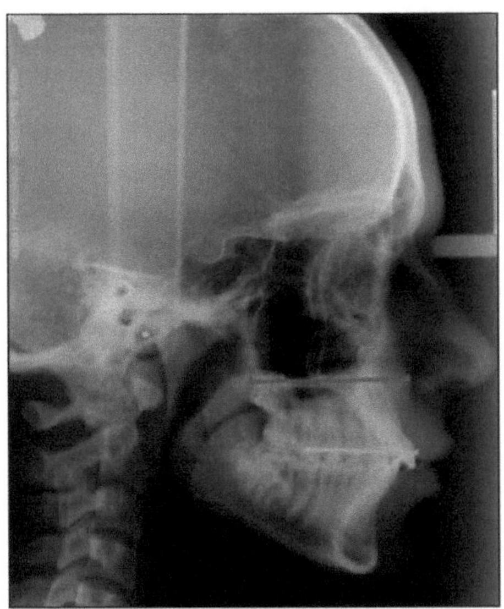

FIGURA 42   - Representative X-ray of the Ena-Enp ratio

Applying the paired t-test before and after orthodontic treatment in group 1 showed a statistically significant difference at the 5% level and assessing the ratio means showed that there was an approximation to the golden number [18] (Figure 36). These findings are in line with those obtained by [15, 28, 97, 104, 111]. With regard to group 2, there was no statistically significant difference at the 5% significance level. Dotto (2006) [24] found that this ratio did not tend to be golden at any stage of growth, neither for females nor for males; however, the author used individuals with Down syndrome as a sample.

When the t-test was applied at a 5% significance level to check for the presence of a golden ratio in both groups, before orthodontic treatment they were not in a golden ratio and after treatment they were not in a golden ratio either. Some authors, when assessing individuals with malocclusion, obtained similar results to ours [7, 8, 20, 79].

The V1S-C1MS segment can suffer variations directly from occlusal disorders, due to the fact that they are horizontal factors contained in the maxilla [46, 96]. By correcting the inadequate dental position, the professional is also helping to bring it closer to the golden number.

Ratio 6 (V1S-C1MS/C1MS-DM16) consists of two segments at tooth points, one segment (V1S-C1MS) and another segment consisting of a point in the V1S tooth region and another point in the distal mandible, at the height of the V1S-C1MS line (C1MS-DM16). This ratio was considered one of the most important for this research project.

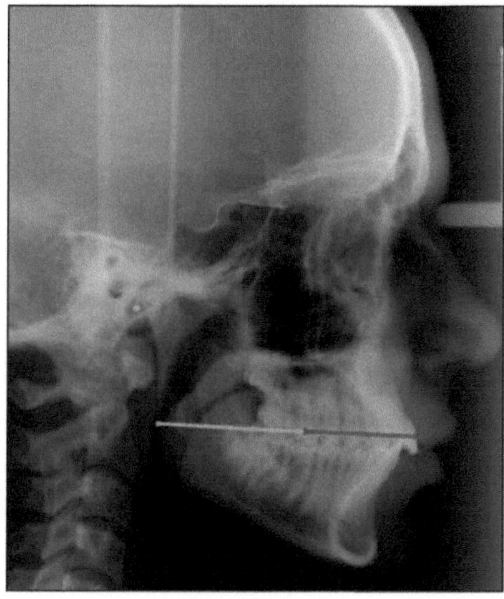

FIGURA 43   - Representative X-ray of the V1S-C1MS/ ratio

In group 1, which was considered to have an aesthetic improvement when compared before and after orthodontic treatment, the paired t-test showed a statistically significant difference at the 5% level and when evaluating the means of the ratio it was observed that there was an approximation in relation to the golden number. The graph (Figure 36) shows a significant approximation in relation to the golden number after orthodontic treatment, a similar result observed by [104]. Castilho (2005) [20] studied this ratio and found no statistically significant difference when comparing before and after orthodontic treatment; however, the sample consisted of individuals undergoing orthopaedic/orthodontic treatment [39]. In group 2, there was no statistically significant difference in the paired t-test compared before and after orthodontic treatment.

When the t-test was applied at a 5% significance level to check for the presence of a golden ratio, group 1 did not have a golden ratio before treatment and after treatment it was found to be in proportion. In group 2, both before and after orthodontic treatment, the ratio was outside the golden ratio and remained outside the golden ratio. According to Langlade (2002) [46], if the upper incisor teeth are too buccalised, this results in a smile showing the gums too much, with a suppressed upper lip, compromising facial harmony and consequently facial aesthetics. However, when compared after orthodontic treatment, where the anterior teeth have a more harmonious conformation, the result is closer to the golden ratio. And because it is a horizontal distance in the region of the teeth, the orthodontist can modify it considerably with treatment [37]. This fact can be confirmed in our research work by analysing the data, in which we observed a statistically significant difference, and comparing before and after treatment we found an approximation in relation to the golden ratio. In addition, the group with aesthetic improvement before treatment did not have a golden ratio and after treatment had a golden ratio

Ratio 7 (Ena-Me/A-B) (Figure 44), the last **ratio** studied in this research project, consists of 2 vertical segments, one relating maxilla and mandible (Ena-Me) and the other also relating maxilla and mandible (A-B).

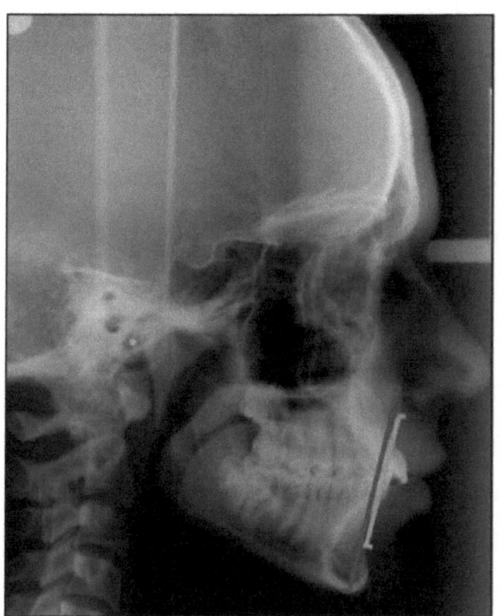

FIGURA 44   - Representative X-ray of the Ena-Me/ ratio

When comparing before and after orthodontic treatment in both groups, there was no statistically significant difference in the paired t-test at the 5% significance level, a similar result observed by [104]. When the t-test was applied at the 5% significance level in order to verify the presence of the golden ratio, in group 1 before treatment the ratio was not in the golden ratio and afterwards it remained outside the golden ratio. Group 2 did not have a golden ratio before orthodontic treatment and had a golden ratio after treatment. According to Interlandi (1999) [37], vertical distances are the most difficult for orthodontists. Nielsen (1991) [69] also reported that mandibular growth is one of the main factors responsible for modifying vertical distances; however, the A-B distance, especially when it comes to point B, can be influenced by orthodontic treatment [37, 64, 82],

This study found that of the 7 ratios studied comparing the two groups: 1) Aesthetic improvement compared before and after orthodontic treatment and 2) No aesthetic improvement compared before and after orthodontic treatment, in **ratio 3** (A-Pog/V1S-C1MS), group 1 showed a statistically significant difference approaching the golden number, while group 2 showed no statistically significant difference. In **ratio 5** (Ena-Enp/V1S-C1MS), there was a similar difference to ratio 3, i.e. group 1 differed in a statistically significant way, coming close to the golden number on average, while group 2 showed no statistically significant difference. In both ratios, it can be seen that group 1, because it was made up of individuals with an aesthetic improvement, the treatment suggests that these ratios should be directed towards the golden number, while in group 2 there was no difference. **Ratio 6** (V1S-C1MS/C1MS-DM16) in group 1 before treatment was not in golden ratio and after treatment was found to be in ratio, however in group 2, both before and after orthodontic treatment the ratio was outside the golden ratio and remained outside the golden ratio. Therefore, in group 1 there were three ratios that differed in a statistically significant way and in group 2 only one ratio differed in a statistically significant way.

The aim of this research study was to delve a little deeper into the study of the golden ratio in order to enrich the literature and clarify its main purpose, which is to promote a tool for individualised analysis of the patient rather than measures based on population averages. In addition, a cephalometric programme was developed for this study, which presents the cephalometric analysis used in this research study, with the aim of contributing to the feasibility of applying the golden ratio in conjunction with other cephalometric analyses.

This opens new doors for further studies and new discoveries on this subject, contributing in some way to the search for patient well-being, satisfaction and joy, one of the main goals that dental professionals should strive for.

CHAPTER 9

CONCLUSIONS

Based on the methodology employed and the analysis of the results obtained, we conclude:

a) in group 1 - improvement after orthodontic treatment: the A-Pog/V1S-C1MS, Ena-Enp/V1S-C1MS and V1S-C1MS/C1MS-DM16 ratios differed in a statistically significant way when comparing before and after orthodontic treatment. The V1S-C1MS/C1MS-DM16 ratio before treatment was not in golden ratio and after treatment it became in golden ratio.

b) in group 2 - there was no improvement after orthodontic treatment: only the N-Ena/V1S-DM16 ratio differed in a statistically significant way when comparing before and after treatment. The A-Pog/V1S-DM16 ratio before treatment was in golden ratio before treatment and after treatment it was not in golden ratio.

REFERENCES

1 Alam MK, Noor NFM, Basri R, Yew TF, Wen TH. Multiracial facial golden ratio and evaluation of facial appearance. PLoS One. 2015; 10 (11): 1-22.

2 Albuquerque Júnior, HR, Almeida MHC. Evaluation of the reproducibility error of cephalometric values applied in the Tweed-Merrifield philosophy, by computerised and conventional methods. Ortodontia. 1998; 31 (3): 18-30.

3 Al-Marzok, Majeed KRA, Ibrahim IK. Evaluation of maxillary anterior teeth and their relation to the Golden proportion in malaysian population. BMC Oral Health 2013; 13:9.

4 Amoric M. The golden number: applications to cranio-facial evaluation. Funct Orthod. 1995 Jan-Feb; 12(1): 18-21,24-5.

5 Andrews LF. The six keys to normal occlusion. Am J Orthod Dentofacial Orthod. 1972 sep; 62 (3): 296-309.

6 Araújo ECCBC Study of the golden ratio using lateral cephalometric radiographs in individuals with normal occlusion who are on the upward curve of the pubertal growth spurt [dissertation]. Master's Degree in Oral Biopathology - Area of Concentration in Dental Radiology - School of Dentistry, São José dos Campos Campus, Universidade Estadual Paulista; 2003.

7 Araújo MM, Passeri LA, Araújo, A. Pre- and post-operative cephalometric analysis of Fibonacci divine ratios in patients undergoing mandibular advancement. Dental Press Ortodon Ortop Facial. 2001 Nov-Dec; 6 (6): 29-36.

8 Baker BW, Woods MG. The role of the divine proportion in the aesthetic improvement of patients undergoing combined orthodontic/orthognathic surgical treatment. Int J Adult Orthodon Orthognath Surg. 2001; 16 (2): 108-20.

9 Barrer J G, Ghafari J. Silhouette profiles in the assessment of facial esthetics: a comparison of cases treated with various orthodontic appliances. Am J Orthod. 1985 May; 87 (5): 385-91.

10Baum AT. Orthodontic treatment and the maturing face. Angle Orthod. 1966Apr; 36 (2): 121-35.

UBenjafield J. The 'golden rectangle': some new data. Am J PsychoL 1976 Dec; 89 (4): 737-43.

12Bertollo RM, Silva DL, Oliveira L, Bergoli RD, Oliveira MG. Evaluation of Facial Harmony in Relation to Fibonacci's Divine Proportions. Rev Port Estomatol Cir Maxilofac. 2008; 49: 213-219.

13Bishara SE *et al.* A Computer assisted photogrammetric analysis of soft tisue changes after orthodontic treatment. Part 1: Methodology and reliability. Am J Orthod Dentofacial Orthop. 1995; 107 (6): 633-9.

14 Bittencourt MAV. Clinical photography in orthodontic practice - Part I: basics and equipment. Rev Soc Odontol Bras. 1999 Jan-Jun; 3(7): 281-4.

15Bragatto FP, Chicarelli M, Kasuya AVB, Takeshita WM, Iwaki-Filho L, Iwaki LCV. Golden Proportion Analysis of Dental-Skeletal Patterns of Class II and III Patients Pre and Post Orthodontic-orthognatic Treatment. The Journal of Contemporary Dental Practice, September 2016; 17(9): 728-733.

16Brangeli LAM *et al.* Comparative study of cephalometric analysis using the manual and computerised methods. Rev Assoe Paul Cir Dent. 2000 May-Jun; 54 (3): 234-41.

17Britton J. Fibonacci number in nature [internet]. Available at: http://britton.disted.camosun.bc.ca/fibslide/ibfibslide.htm. Accessed on 10 Oct 2006.

18Brum CVA, Saltori FA, Silva MCP, Pereira AC, Cunha FL, Paranhos LR. Study of the golden ratio in young Class II, division q patients treated orthodontically. Odonto. 2010; 18 (35): 70-80.

19Burstone CJ. The integumental profile. Am J Orthod. 1958 Jan; 44 (1): 1-25.

20 Castilho JCM. Verification of the golden ratio in individuals at the beginning and end of orthopaedic/orthodontic treatment using cephalometric radiographs [thesis]. Associate Professor in Dental Radiology -

School of Dentistry, Universidade Estadual Paulista, São José dos Campos; 2005.

21 Claman L, Patton D, Rashid R. Standardised portrait photography for dental patients. Am J Orthod Dentofacial Orthop. 1990 Sep; 98 (3): 197- 205.

22 Colombo VL *et al.* Frontal facial analysis at rest and during smiling in standardised photographs. Part I - Evaluation at rest, Rev Dent Press Orthod Orthop. 2004 May-Jun; 9 (3): 47-58.

23 Czarnecki ST, Nanda RS, Currier GF. Perceptions of a balanced facial profile. Am J Orthod Dentofacial Orthop. 1993 Aug; 104 (2): 180-7.

24Dotto PP. Verification of the golden ratio in lateral cephalometric measurements of individuals with Down syndrome [thesis]. PhD in Oral Biopathology - Area of Concentration in Dental Radiology) - School of Dentistry, Universidade Estadual Paulista, São José dos Campos; 2006.

25 Eduardo JVP. Study of the vertical dimension of occlusion and plane of orientation applying the golden ratio [thesis]. Doctorate in Dentistry - Area of Concentration in Prosthodontics) - Faculty of Dentistry, University of São Paulo, São Paulo; 2000.

26 Ferraz H. Systems of mathematical proportions. Rev Eletrónica. 2004 Apr; 26: 1-10. Available at :

http://www.cdcc.sc.usp.br/ciencia/artigos/art_26/proporcao.html. Accessed on: 10 Oct 2006.

27 Garbin AJL Analysis of fibonacci divine ratios in lateral teleradiographs of patients with normal occlusion [dissertation]. Master's Degree in Orthodontics - Piracicaba School of Dentistry, State University of Campinas, Piracicaba; 1997.

28 Garbin AJL Analysis of divine proportions in lateral teleradiographs of patients submitted to mandibular retropositioning surgery [thesis]. PhD in Orthodontics - Piracicaba School of Dentistry, State University of Campinas, Piracicaba; 1999.

29 Ghyka M. The geometry of life. In. The geometry of art and life. New York: Dover; 1977. Chap.6, p.87-110.

30 Gil CTLA. Study of the golden ratio in the skull architecture of individuals with normal occlusion, based on lateral, frontal and axial teleradiographs [thesis]. Doctorate in Dentistry - Area of Concentration in Dental Radiology - School of Dentistry, Universidade Estadual Paulista, São José dos Campos; 1999.

31 Gil CTLA. Craniofacial golden ratio. São Paulo: Santos; 2001.100p.

32 Gil CTLA, Mediei Filho E. Study of the golden ratio in the craniofacial architecture of adult individuals with normal occlusion, based on axial, frontal and lateral teleradiographies. Ortodontia. 2002 Apr-Jun; 35: 69-85.

33 Goldsman S. The variations in skeletal and denture patterns in excellent adult facial types. Angle Orthod. 1959 Apr; 29 (2).

34 Halazonetis DJ. Computer-assisted cephalometric analysis. Am J Orthod Dentofacial Orthop. 1994 May; 105 (5): 517-21.

35 Houston WJB. The analysis of errors in orthodontic measurements. Am J Orthod. 1983 May; 83 (5): 382-90.

36 Howells DJ, Shaw WC. The validity and reability of ratings of dental and facial attractiveness for epidemiologic use. Am J Orthod. 1985 Nov; 88 (5): 402-8.

37 Interlandi S. Ortodontia: bases para a iniciação 4.ed. São Paulo: Artes Médicas; 1999.769p.

38 Jacobson A. Radiographic cephalometry: from basics to videoimaging. Chicago: Quintessence; 1995. 322p.

39 Jahanbin A, Poosti M, Salari S, Esmaily H, Sagha H. Effect of changes in divine proportion on aesthetic perception of smile in frontal view. J Craniofac Surg. 2013; 24 (6): 1946-9.

40 Jefferson Y. Skeletal types: key to unravelling the mystery of facial beauty and its biologic significance. J General Orthod. 1996 Jun; 7 (2): 7-25.

41 Jeferson Y. Facial beauty [internet]. Available at: http://www.facialbeautv.org. Accessed on: 19 December 2003.

42 Kerr WJS, O'donnel JM. Panei perception of facial attractiveness. Br J Orthod. 1990 Nov; 17 (4): 299-304.

43 Knott R. Fibonacci number and golden section [internet]. Available at:

http://www.mcs.surrey.ac.Uk/Personal/R.Knott/Fibonacci/fibnat.html. Accessed on: 18 April 2006.

44Kõller GL The growth, development and maturation of the face: a contemporary view [Internet]. Available at: http://www.spo.orq.br/qerson.html. Accessed on: 18 Apr. 2006.

45Landgraf ME *et al.* Facial analysis, a key element in contemporary orthodontic diagnosis. Orthodontics. 2002 Apr; 35 (2): 147-159.

46Langlade M. Diagnóstico ortodontico 2.ed. São Paulo: Ed. Santos, 2002. 742p.

47Levin E. The golden proportion, beauty and dental aesthetics [internet]. Available at: http://qoldenmeanqauqe.co.uk. Accessed on: 18 Apr. 2006.

48Levin El. Dental aesthetics and golden proportion. J Prosthet Dent. 1978 Sep; 40 (3): 244-251.

49Loffredo LCM. Study of the reproducibility of information in the health area [thesis]. Livre Docência Universidade Estadual Paulista Júlio de Mesquita Filho. - School of Dentistry, São Paulo State University, Araraquara; 1996.

50Lombardi RE. The principies of visual perception and their clinical application to denture esthetics. J Prosthet Dent. 1972 Apr; 29 (4): 358- 82.

51 Lopes Filho JA, Silva SS. Anthropometry: on man as an integral part of environmental factors. Its functionality, scope and use [Internet]. Available at   :
http://www.vitruvius.com.br/arquitextos/arq000/esp204.asp. Accessed on:

10 October 2006.

52 Machado AW, Souki BQ. Simplifying the acquisition and use of digital images - scanners and digital cameras. Rev Dent Press Ortod Ortop. 2004 Jul/Aug; 9 (4): 133-56.

53 Machado CR. Photography in Orthodontics. Ortodontia. 1974 Jan-Apr; 7 (1): 3-18.

54 Mack MR. Perspective of facial aesthetics in dental treatment planning. J Prosthet Dent. 1996 Feb; 75 (2): 169-76 (Review).

55 Marinho Filho AV, Teramoto L, Andrade NJ. Divine proportion - Cephalometrics and Art? Ortodontia. 1982 Jan-Apr; 15 (1): 35-9.

56 Marquadt S. The facial masks [internet]. Available at: http://www.beautyanalysis.com/index2_mba.htm. Accessed on: 10 Oct 2006.

57 Martins LP *et al*. Reproducibility error of Steiner and Ricketts cephalometric analysis measurements by conventional and computerised methods. Ortodontia. 1995 Jan-Apr; 28 (1): 4-17.

58 Martins MV. Evaluation of the golden ratio in individuals with normal occlusion using lateral cephalometric radiographs [dissertation]. Master's Degree in Oral Biopathology Area of Concentration - Dental Radiology - School of Dentistry, Universidade Estadual Paulista, São José dos Campos; 2003.

59 Martins MV. Study of equalities and golden ratios in craniofacial

measurements using lateral cephalometric radiographs [thesis]. PhD in Oral Biopathology Area of Concentration - Dental Radiology - School of Dentistry, Universidade Estadual Paulista, São José dos Campos; 2005.

60Meisner G. The evolution of truth [internet]. Available at: http:// www.qoldennumber.net. Accessed on: 19 December 2003.

61 Mew J. Suggestions for forecasting and monitoring facial growth. Am J Orthod Dentofac Orthop. 1993 Aug; 104 (2): 105-20.

62Michiels G, Sather AH. Validity and reliability of facial profile evaluation in vertical and horizontal dimensions from lateral cephalograms and lateral photographs. Int J Adult Orthod Orthognath Surg. 1994 Jan; 9 (1): 43-54.

63 Miquilito JL. Comparison of the results obtained between three methods, one manual and two computerised, of angular and linear values in lateral cephalometric radiographs [thesis]. PhD

Dentistry - School of Dentistry, Universidade Estadual Paulista, São José dos Campos; 2003.

64Moyers RE. Orthodontics 4ª Ed. Rio de Janeiro: Guanabara Koogan; 1991. 483p.

65Nakajima E, Yanagisawa M. The Japanese sense of beauty and facial proportions. The facial characteristics of people with malocclusion. Quintessence Int.1985; 16 (8): 553-7.

66Nakajima E, Maeda T, Yanagisawa M. The Japanese sense of beauty and facial proportions. The beautiful face and the A/2 rule. Quintessence Int.

1985; 16(9): 629-37.

67Netto L. Segmento áureo aplicado à construções de violoncelos e violinos [internet]. Disponível: http://members.tripod.com/caraipora/proporouro.htm. Accessed on: 12 Dec. 2003.

68 Nguyen MS, Saag M, Le VN, Jagomagi TTNT. The golden proportion in facial soft-tissues of Vietnamese females. Stomatologija, Baltic Dental and Maxillofacial Journal. 2016; 18 (3): 80-85.

69Nielsen IL. Vertical malocclusions: etiology, development, diagnosis and some aspects of treatment. Angle Orthod. 1991 Winter; 61 (4): 247-60. Review.

70Okuyama CC, Martins DR. Preference of the integumentary facial profile in young leucoderm, melanoderm and xanthoderm men of both sexes.

sexes, evaluated by orthodontists, laypeople and visual artists. Orthodontics.1997; 30 (1): 6-19.

71Oliveira Júnior OB. Smile builders - science or art? APCD São José do Rio Preto [internet]. Available at: http://www.apcdriopreto.com.br/artiqos2.asp?codiqo=6. Accessed on: 10 Oct 2006.

72Ono E. Study of the golden ratio in brachial and mesofacial individuals using lateral cephalometric radiographs [dissertation]. Master's Degree in Oral Biopathology - Area of Concentration in Dental Radiology - School of Dentistry, Universidade Estadual Paulista, São José dos Campos; 2005.

73 Packiriswamy V, Kumar P, Rao M. Identification of Facial Shape by Applying Golden Ratio to the Facial Measurements: An Interracial Study in Malaysian Population. N Am J Med Sei. 2012 Dec; 4 (12): 624-629.

74 Peck H, Peck S. A concept of facial estheties. Angle Orthod. 1970 Oct; 40 (4): 284-319.

75 Peerlings RH, Kuijpers-Jagtman, A, Hoeskma JBA. Photographic scale to measure facial aesthetics. Eur J Orthod. 1995; 17: 101-9.

76 Petronzelli C. Golden division [internet]. Available at: http://www.expoente.com.br/professores/kalinke/projeto/aurea.htm. Accessed on: 10 October 2006.

77 Piccin MR. Verification of the divine proportion of the face in fully dentate patients [dissertation]. Master's Degree in Physiology and Biophysics of the Stomatognathic System - Piracicaba School of Dentistry, State University of Campinas, Piracicaba; 1997.

78 Piehl J. The golden section: the "true" ratio? Percept Mot Skill. 1978 Jun; 46 (3): 831-4.

79 Piselli LGO. Application of the golden ratio in the vertical and horizontal assessment of Class II, 1st division patients undergoing orthodontic treatment [dissertation]. Master's Degree in Dental Radiology - Piracicaba School of Dentistry, State University of Campinas, Piracicaba; 2003.

80 Powell SJ, Rayson RK. The profile in facial aesthetics. Br J Orthod. 1976 Oct; 3 (4): 207-15.

81 Preston JD. The golden proportion revisited. J Esthet Dent.1993 Aug; 5 (6): 247-51.

82 Proffit WR, Sields Júnior HW. Contemporary orthodontics 2.ed. Rio de Janeiro: Guanabara Koogan; 1995.

83 Rakosi T, Jonas I, Graber TM. Orthodontics and facial orthopaedics. Porto Alegre: Artmed; 1999.

84Ranulfo AA. Traditional Freemasonry I [Internet] Available at: http://www.qeocities.com/templosalomao/eqipcios.htm. Accessed on: 10 Oct 2006

85Ricketts RM. Planning treatment on the basic of the facial pattern and estimate of its growth. Angle Orthod. 1957; 27 (1): 14-37.

86Ricketts RM. A principie of partial growth of the mandible. Angle Orthod.1972 Oct; 42 (4): 366-8.

87Ricketts RM. The golden divider. J Clin Orthod. 1981 Nov; 15 (11): 752-9.

88Ricketts RM. The biologic significance of the divine proportion and Fibonacci series. Am J Orthod. 1982May; 81 (5): 351-70.

89Riedel RA. Esthetics and its relation to orthodontic therapy. Angle Orthod. 1950 Jul; 20 (3): 168-78.

90Riedel RA. An analysis of dento facial relationships. Am J Orthod. 1957 Feb; 43 (2): 103-19.

91 Rufenacht CR. Fundamentals of aesthetics. São Paulo: Ed. Santos, Quintessence; 1998. 375p.

92 Santos JE. Study of the golden ratio in facial photographs of individuals with normal occlusion [dissertation]. Master's Degree in Orthodontics - Methodist University of São Paulo School of Dentistry, Methodist University of São Paulo, São Bernardo do Campo; 2003.

93 Santos SH. Application of the linear and geometric method using lateral cephalometric radiographs to differentiate and identify the divine proportion in the three facial types: mesofacial, brachyfacial and dolichofacial [thesis]. PhD in Oral Biopathology - Area of Concentration in Dental Radiology - School of Dentistry, Universidade Estadual Paulista, São José dos Campos; 2004.

94 Scolozzi P, Momjian A, Courvoisier D. Dentofacial Deformities Treated According to a Dentoskeletal Analysis Based on the Divine Proportion: Are the Resulting Faces de Facto "Divinely" Proportioned? J Craniofac Surg2011;22: 147-150.

95 Shinozaki EB. Facial analysis [monograph] Specialisation Course in Orthodontics, School of Dentistry - School of Dentistry, Universidade Estadual Paulista, São José dos Campos; 2000.

96 Silva MAS. Study of the divine proportion in the skull architecture of individuals with Angle Class II occlusion, based on lateral cephalometric radiographs [dissertation]. Master's Degree in Oral Biopathology - Area of Concentration in Dental Radiology - School of Dentistry, Universidade Estadual Paulista, São José dos Campos; 2003.

97 Silva MAS. Evaluation of the divine craniofacial proportion before and after orthodontic treatment, in photographs and lateral cephalometric radiographs [thesis]. PhD in Oral Biopathology - Area of concentration in Dental Radiology - School of Dentistry, Universidade Estadual Paulista, São José dos Campos; 2005.

98 Snow SR. Esthetic smile analysis of maxillary anterior tooth width: the golden percentage. J Esthet Dent.1999; 11 (4): 177-84.

99 Sodré U, Toffoli SFL. Essential maths: Fibonacci sequences, various applications . Available at : http://pessoal.sercomtel.com.br/matematica/aleqria/fibon/seqfib2.htm#fib 31. Accessed on: 12 December 2003.

100 Souza HRMC *et al.* Geometry applied to Greek art [internet]. Available at: http://www.pro.ufjf.br/desqeo/Trabalhos/Art TOGS.pdf. Accessed on 10 Oct 2006.

101 Spyropoulos MN, Halazonetis DJ. Significance of the tissue profile on facial esthetics. Am J Orthod Orthop. 2001 May; 119 (5): 464-71.

102 Stoner MM. A photometric analysis of the facila profile. Am J Orthod. 1955 Jun; 41 (6): 453-469.

103 Suguino R *et al.* Facial analysis. Rev Dent Press Orthod Orthop. 1996 Sep-Oct; 1 (1): 86-107.

104 Takeshita WM. Verification of the golden ratio in lateral cephalometric radiographs of Angle Class II patients before and after orthodontic treatment [dissertation]. Master's Degree in the Postgraduate Programme in Oral

Biopathology - Dental Radiology - São José dos Campos School of Dentistry, São José dos Campos State University, São José dos Campos; 2004.

105 Tavares EO *et al.* The proportion of geometric schemes in Renaissance painting [Internet]; 2002. Available at: http://www.pro.ufif.br/desqeo/Trabalhos/Art_Tavares.pdf. Accessed on: 10 Oct 2006.

106 Toniello PT, Silva MC, Iwaki LCV, Gisette M. Divine proportion in individuals with skeletal occlusions I, II and III in lateral cephalometric radiographs. Rev. Cubana EstomatoL 2014;51(2):132-144.

107 Torres R. Harmonious growth and divine proportion. Divulg Cult Odontol. 1970 Mar-Apr; 162:3-13.

108 Trevisan F. Photogrammetric and subjective analysis of the facial profile of young Brazilian men with normal occlusion [dissertation]. Master's Degree in Orthodontics - Methodist University of São Paulo School of Dentistry, Methodist University of São Paulo, São Bernardo do Campo; 2003.

109 Vedovello SAS. et al. Facial analysis: study of lateral proportions. Orthodontics.2001 May-Aug; 34 (2): 81-5.

110 Vegter F, Hage JJ. Clinicai anthropometry and canons of the face in historical perspective. Plast Recontr Surg. 2000 Oct; 106 (5): 1090-6.

111 Walewski LA. et al. Analysis of the facial skeletal and soft tissue profile

before and after orthognathic surgery in Class II and III patients, and its relationship with the golden ratio. Rev Odontol UNESP. 2017 Sep-Oct; 46 (5): 292-298.

112 Walter-porto CO. Evaluation of the Golden Ratio in dolichofacial and mesofacial individuals using lateral cephalometric radiographs [dissertation] Master's Degree in Oral Biopathology - Area of Expertise

concentration in Dental Radiology) - School of Dentistry, Universidade Estadual Paulista, São José dos Campos; 2005.

113 Wuerpel EH. The inspiration of beauty. Angle Orthod. 1932 Oct; 2 (4): 201-18.

114 Wuerpel EH. On facial balance and harmony. Angle Orthod. 1937 Jan; 7(1): 81-9.

115 Zietsman ST, Wiltshire WA, Coetzee CE. The Divine Proportion and the cranial base. J Dent Res. 1997; 76 (5): 1202. (Abstract).

116 Zietsman ST, Wiltshire WA, Greeff C. The Golden proportion in cephalometrics. J Dent Res. 1995; 74 (3): 1020, 1995. (Abstract).

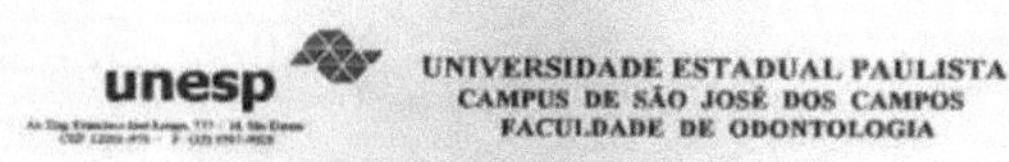

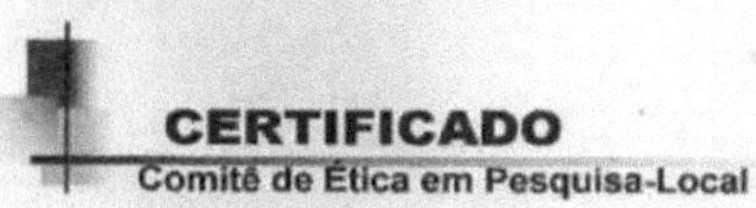

CERTIFICADO

Comitê de Ética em Pesquisa-Local

CERTIFICAMOS, que o protocolo n° 046/2005-PH/CEP, sobre "Verificação da relação entre proporção áurea e estética facial, antes e depois do tratamento ortodôntico, utilizando radiografias cefalométricas laterais e fotografias, sob a responsabilidade de WILTON MITSUNARI TAKESHITA, está de acordo com os Princípios Éticos, seguindo diretrizes e normas regulamentadoras de pesquisa, envolvendo seres humanos, conforme Resolução n° 196/96 do Conselho Nacional de Saúde e foi aprovado pelo Comitê de Ética em Pesquisa.

São José dos Campos, 13 de setembro de 2005.

____

Profa. Dra. Suely Carvalho Mutti Naressi
Coordenadora do Comitê de Ética em Pesquisa-Local

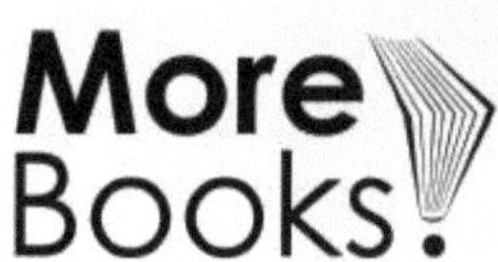

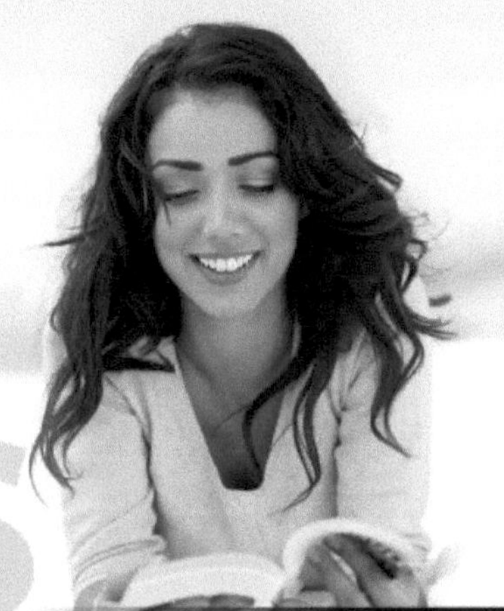

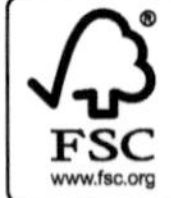

Printed by Books on Demand GmbH, Norderstedt / Germany